Sara Hutchison

# Physical and Cognitive Training in Old Age

Sara Hutchison

# Physical and Cognitive Training in Old Age

Intervention Effects on Cognition and Well-Being

Südwestdeutscher Verlag für Hochschulschriften

**Impressum/Imprint (nur für Deutschland/ only for Germany)**
Bibliografische Information der Deutschen Nationalbibliothek: Die Deutsche Nationalbibliothek verzeichnet diese Publikation in der Deutschen Nationalbibliografie; detaillierte bibliografische Daten sind im Internet über http://dnb.d-nb.de abrufbar.
Alle in diesem Buch genannten Marken und Produktnamen unterliegen warenzeichen-, markenoder patentrechtlichem Schutz bzw. sind Warenzeichen oder eingetragene Warenzeichen der jeweiligen Inhaber. Die Wiedergabe von Marken, Produktnamen, Gebrauchsnamen, Handelsnamen, Warenbezeichnungen u.s.w. in diesem Werk berechtigt auch ohne besondere Kennzeichnung nicht zu der Annahme, dass solche Namen im Sinne der Warenzeichen- und Markenschutzgesetzgebung als frei zu betrachten wären und daher von jedermann benutzt werden dürften.

Verlag: Südwestdeutscher Verlag für Hochschulschriften Aktiengesellschaft & Co. KG
Dudweiler Landstr. 99, 66123 Saarbrücken, Deutschland
Telefon +49 681 37 20 271-1, Telefax +49 681 37 20 271-0, Email: info@svh-verlag.de
Zugl.: Bern, Universität Bern, Inauguraldissertation, 2008

Herstellung in Deutschland:
Schaltungsdienst Lange o.H.G., Berlin
Books on Demand GmbH, Norderstedt
Reha GmbH, Saarbrücken
Amazon Distribution GmbH, Leipzig
ISBN: 978-3-8381-0539-0

**Imprint (only for USA, GB)**
Bibliographic information published by the Deutsche Nationalbibliothek: The Deutsche Nationalbibliothek lists this publication in the Deutsche Nationalbibliografie; detailed bibliographic data are available in the Internet at http://dnb.d-nb.de.
Any brand names and product names mentioned in this book are subject to trademark, brand or patent protection and are trademarks or registered trademarks of their respective holders. The use of brand names, product names, common names, trade names, product descriptions etc. even without a particular marking in this works is in no way to be construed to mean that such names may be regarded as unrestricted in respect of trademark and brand protection legislation and could thus be used by anyone.

Publisher:
Südwestdeutscher Verlag für Hochschulschriften Aktiengesellschaft & Co. KG
Dudweiler Landstr. 99, 66123 Saarbrücken, Germany
Phone +49 681 37 20 271-1, Fax +49 681 37 20 271-0, Email: info@svh-verlag.de

Copyright © 2009 by the author and Südwestdeutscher Verlag für Hochschulschriften Aktiengesellschaft & Co. KG and licensors
All rights reserved. Saarbrücken 2009

Printed in the U.S.A.
Printed in the U.K. by (see last page)
ISBN: 978-3-8381-0539-0

# 1 INTRODUCTION .................................................................................................................. 3

# 2 CHALLENGES AND OPPORTUNITIES OF OLD AGE ............................................. 5
2.1 CHANGES IN THE AGING BODY ......................................................................................... 6
2.2 CHANGES IN THE AGING BRAIN ....................................................................................... 10
2.3 AGE-ASSOCIATED ILLNESSES AND COMORBIDITY ........................................................... 13
2.4 PERSONALITY DEVELOPMENT IN OLD AGE ...................................................................... 14
2.5 AGE-ASSOCIATED CHANGES IN COGNITION ..................................................................... 16
2.6 A SPECIAL CHALLENGE: MAINTAINING WELL-BEING IN OLD AGE .................................... 23

# 3 HOW TO DEAL WITH THE CHALLENGES OF WELL-BEING AND COGNITION IN OLD AGE: EFFECTS OF INTERVENTION STUDIES ............................................. 33
3.1 PHYSICAL TRAINING EFFECTS ON COGNITION IN OLD AGE .............................................. 33
3.2 COGNITIVE TRAINING EFFECTS ON COGNITION IN OLD AGE ............................................ 38
3.3 COMPARISON OF PHYSICAL AND COGNITIVE TRAINING EFFECTS ON COGNITION ............. 44
3.4 PHYSICAL EXERCISE EFFECTS ON WELL-BEING ............................................................... 46
3.5 COGNITIVE TRAINING EFFECTS ON WELL-BEING ............................................................. 50
3.6 COMPARISON OF PHYSICAL AND COGNITIVE TRAINING EFFECTS ON WELL-BEING ........... 51
3.7 RATIONALE FOR THE PSYCHOLOGICAL INTERVENTION IN EXTRA .................................... 52

# 4 METHOD ........................................................................................................................... 57
4.1 DESIGN .......................................................................................................................... 57
4.2 SAMPLE ......................................................................................................................... 58
4.3 DESCRIPTION OF THE INTERVENTIONS ............................................................................ 61
COGNITIVE TRAINING ............................................................................................................ 61
ECCENTRIC TRAINING ............................................................................................................ 66
CONVENTIONAL STRENGTH TRAINING ................................................................................... 68
4.4 ASSESSMENT .................................................................................................................. 69
4.4.1 COGNITIVE MEASURES ............................................................................................... 71
4.4.2 WELL-BEING MEASURES ............................................................................................ 74
4.5 STATISTICAL ANALYSES ................................................................................................. 77
4.6 HYPOTHESES .................................................................................................................. 78
4.6.1 HYPOTHESES CONCERNED WITH COGNITION .............................................................. 78
4.6.2 HYPOTHESES CONCERNED WITH WELL-BEING ............................................................ 80

# 5 RESULTS .......................................................................................................................... 81
5.1 COGNITION .................................................................................................................... 82
5.1.1 DESCRIPTIVES, DISTRIBUTION TESTING, CORRELATIONS ........................................... 82
5.1.2 HYPOTHESIS TESTING ................................................................................................. 90
5.1.3 SUMMARY OF COGNITIVE RESULTS ........................................................................... 102
5.2 WELL-BEING ................................................................................................................ 104
5.2.1 DESCRIPTIVES, DISTRIBUTION TESTING, CORRELATIONS ......................................... 104
5.2.2 HYPOTHESIS TESTING ............................................................................................... 109
5.2.3 SUMMARY OF WELL-BEING RESULTS ........................................................................ 115

# 6 DISCUSSION .................................................................................................................. 116

# REFERENCES .................................................................................................................... 123

*"Age is a question of mind over matter. If you don't mind, it doesn't matter."*
—Satchel Paige


*"Nobody grows old merely by living a number of years. We grow old by deserting our ideals. Years may wrinkle the skin, but to give up enthusiasm wrinkles the soul."*
—Samuel Ullman

# 1 Introduction

The life stage of old age is gaining in societal importance, as the percentage of old people in our society increases. In 1900, only 0.5% of the Swiss population were older than 80. In 2003, this number had risen to 4.4% (Swiss Federal Office of Statistics, 2005). The increasing number of old people is due partly to a higher life expectancy and decreasing birth rates. Other crucial factors are improved health management, a higher standard of living and improved work conditions. Especially these second factors have led to a marked increase in the years of later life (Grundy & Bowling, 1999). This demographic development is far from finished – the number of old people will continue to grow, while the number of young people will diminish further. To illustrate, the populous baby boom cohort (i.e. people born between 1946 and 1964) is now middle-aged and has yet to reach old age. Therefore, the percentage of over 65 year olds (of the total population) is expected to stabilize only around the year 2035. Until then, it is expected that the ratio of old to young people will continue to grow.

Switzerland is not the only country whose demographics are changing in the way described above. Germany, France, Italy, the Netherlands, Austria, Sweden or the United Kingdom are examples of european countries facing similar changes. Worldwide there is a trend for a percentual increase of the over 65 year olds. This trend is stronger in the more developed regions (Lehr, 2003). Not only the life expectancy has increased - people also tend to be in good health up to a later point in life than a few decades ago (compression of morbidity, Fries, 2005); they are therefore also able to participate in a wide range of activities up to a much older age than used to be the case.

From all this, it becomes apparent that old age will play an increasingly big role in society and in the life of individuals in the years to come. It is thus doubly important to „add life to years and not just years to life". This is important from an economical, medical as well as from a psychological and ethical standpoint. The question, of course, is how this aim can be achieved. How can the quality of life, the well-being and the cognitive functioning of the elderly be improved?

This thesis aims to shed light on that topic by first examining changes, challenges and opportunities associated with aging. Seeing as physical and cognitive fitness have been shown to be important factors in the quality of life in the elderly, and on the basis of a resource model of well-being, results from an interdisciplinary intervention study employing physical and cognitive training will be presented.

This intervention study, called ExTrA, is primarily concerned with reducing the likelihood of falls in the elderly. ExTrA stands for „eccentric training with the elderly" (in german, *Ex*zentrisches *Tr*aining für *Ä*ltere). It is an interdisciplinary project from the Swiss National Science Foundation program "musculosceletal health - chronic pain" (NFP 53[1]), headed by Prof. Hans Hoppeler from the Institute of Anatomy and Prof. Walter Perrig from the Institute of Psychology of the University of Bern, in collaboration with P. Perrig-Chiello, University of Bern, S.L. Lindstedt, University of Northern Arizona, Flagstaff, USA, and A. Schneider and H. Thüler, BASPO, Switzerland.

A new type of training paradigm, chronic eccentric exercise, was proposed to improve lower limb strength and muscle coordination in the elderly. Traditional trainings are usually based on concentric muscle training, i.e. the training focusses on muscle contraction. Eccentric muscle training, in contrast, denotes training while the muscle is lengthening. As eccentric muscle work places high demands on coordination (more than concentric training), considerable cognitive control is needed. It was therefore hypothesized that eccentric exercise would not only increase muscle strength and muscle coordination, but would also lead to an improvement in cognitive performance. To test this hypothesis, 38 participants (all over 75 years old) were assigned to one of three training groups, which trained twice a week for three months. The first group did an eccentric strength training. A second group performed conventional lower limb resistance exercises ("active controls"), while a third group participated in a cognitive training ("inactive controls"). From a psychological point of view, the following questions were central to the study: Will eccentric exercise have the same positive effect on well-being and certain cognitive measures observed for other exercise regimens? Is a cognitive training more effective in enhancing cognitive function than a physical training? Which training will lead to the greatest improvement in well-being, and which one will be most successful in improving cognitive function? Last but least, it will also be of interest to find out whether the cognitive training will yield transfer effects on non-trained cognitive functions.

The answers to these questions should contribute to the knowledge of how well-being and cognitive function in old age can be optimized through specific intervention programs.

---

[1] Project number 4049-405340-104718/1

## 2  Challenges and Opportunities of Old Age

Growing old brings a multitude of challenges. Many people experience during that life stage the loss of loved ones; some people have to leave their homes and move into assisted living; some experience chronic illnesses or increased frailty, others cognitive decline.

However, growing old is also a life-stage that is characterized by increasing inter-individual differences. Older people are a very heterogeneous group, be it in regard to health, functional autonomy or psychological variables (Voelcker-Rehage, Godde, & Staudinger, 2006). Aging does not just harbor challenges, but also opportunities. A sizeable amount of older people maintains a high level of functioning until very old age (Smith & Baltes, 1996); in many others, it is only certain areas of functioning that are affected by an age-associated decline. In sum, old age is a time of increased inter-individual and intra-individual variance. Gerontological research has shown that age-associated losses increase markedly after the age of 80 (e.g. loss of autonomy, Perrig & Perrig-Chiello, 1999, p. 78). In comparison to younger old people, which are still largely autonomous and healthy, the age group of the over 80 year olds (termed oldest-old) is characterized by heightened vulnerabilty and frailty, displaying higher levels of comorbidity and institutionalization as well as a greater usage of medical and care services (Smith, Borchelt, Maier, & Jopp, 2002).

From all this, it should be clear that the term "age-associated" can be misleading, as clearly chronological age is not the sole determinant of physical and psychological functioning in old age, and aging is different for every single person. Nevertheless, to give a picture of what can be expected in "average aging", the following passages will give an overview over changes in the aging body and brain as well as over age-associated illnesses and multimorbidity. However, research has shown that physical aspects alone cannot give a full picture of what aging entails. How a person reacts to the physical changes, despairing or taking it as an opportunity, can make an enormous difference in how old age is experienced. For this reason, personality development in old age will also be covered.

## 2.1 Changes in the aging body

*Age-related declines in the senses*

Vision usually declines with advancing age. Stereooptic vision, photopic sensitivity, color discrimination, acuity as well as contrast sensitivity decrease in old age, while glare sensitivity increases (for a detailed description of changes in vision with aging see Fozard & Gordon-Salant, 2001). Hearing problems also become more frequent with age. One cause of this may be a loss of hair cells in the cochlea, another a loss of neurons comprising the auditory nerve, which leads to reduced afferent transmission of acoustic signals. Furthermore, there is also a reduction in the number of neurons in the auditory nuclei of the brain stem, which may affect acoustic stimulus processing. Last but not least, there are changes in the neurotransmitter system with age, which may cause an increase in neural noise or a reduction in suppression of external noise (Fozard & Gordon-Salant, 2001). A common complaint of older people is also that their sense of smell deteriorates. This may be caused by a loss of olfactory receptor cells or by a change in the composition of the nasal mucus. There may also be detrimental age-effects on the olfactory pathways in the brain. However, it appears that part of the deterioration is due to chronic diseases, medications or other age-reated health issues, and may therefore be limited to a small subsample of the elderly population. The gustatory sense depends to a large degree on smell and is thus also affected by the above-mentioned age-associated decrease of smell.

In summary, most old people will experience an age-related decline in one or more of their senses, thus making sensory decline one of the challenges of old age.

*Age-related declines in muscle mass and motor control*
With advancing age, a loss of muscle mass occurs, causing a steady reduction in physical strength (Bee & Bjorklund, 2004). The most rapid decline starts to occur after the age of fifty. This loss concerns mainly the type II muscle fibres responsible for fast contractions; thus, it is especially in situations demanding fast muscle contractions that this muscle loss becomes apparent. Several studies have also reported a loss of proprioception in old age, i.e. older adults have „reduced joint position sense" (Ketcham & Stelmach, 2001). Another aspect of motor control that is affected by age is movement control. The time to initiate a movement response as well as the actual movement speed are reduced in older people. Furthermore, force production and force regulation decreases (for a more detailed review of age-related declines in motor control see Ketcham & Stelmach 2001). Range of motion and flexibility is usually also decreased. If one considers the combined effects of these factors, it becomes apparent that the ability to make quick and exact movements is reduced in old age. Apart from the loss of muscle fibres there are certain changes in the brain that may account for these problems, e.g. age-related decline of neurons in the basal ganglia, the cerebellum and the motor cortex. Age-related changes in the brain will be discussed in more detail in the next section. The changes in motor control are most obvious from the outside in posture and gait. Older people tend to have a less stable posture and more problems with balance than younger people. They usually take shorter steps and walk slower. Part of this is due to the aspects of motor control already mentioned above. However, postural stability is also dependent on attentional processes, which are also affected by aging (Brown, Shumway-Cook, & Woollacott, 1999).

Problems with balance coupled with reduced proprioception, attention and the inability to create force and speed lead to situations when a stumble cannot be compensated for by a quick compensatory movement. A fall results. About one-third of all people older than 65 falls at least once a year (Walter, Schneider, & Bisson, 2006); for the over 80 year olds, it is already every second person (Stuck, 2003). In addition to all that, people older than 75 years are eleven times more likely to be hospitalized after a fall than 60-64 year olds (Scuffham, Chaplin, & Legood, 2003). A decrease in bone mineral density and the loss of muscle mass and control (sarcopenia) promote fall-related fractures. It becomes therefore clear that for the elderly, a fall is more likely to have grave consequences than for younger adults. It may go as far as to seriously impair an older person's autonomy. A physical training which increases muscle strength and control, as is proposed for eccentric training, could therefore reduce the incidence of falls and fractures in the elderly and help maintain an independent lifestyle.

*Functional autonomy in old age*

Functional autonomy refers to the capability of mastering one's everyday life without outside help (Perrig-Chiello, Staehelin, & Perrig, 1999, p. 20). Functional autonomy is therefore akin to independent living. A crucial component of independent living is to master the everyday activities of daily living (ADL), such as as dressing and personal hygiene. These activities can be considered the basic building blocks of an autonomous life. However, to be truly autonomous one has also to master more complex competencies (usually termed instrumental activities of daily living or IADL), such as shopping and overseeing financial matters, which are in contrast to the ADL more culturally influenced and less automatized. Some researchers go even further and include capabilities such as social and leisure activities as crucial aspects of autonomy (Baltes, Maas, Wims, & Borchelt, 1996).

As is typical for old age, there are great individual differences in the extent of autonomous living in the elderly, even though an age-related deterioration in functional autonomy is a fact (Perrig-Chiello, Perrig, Uebelbacher, & Staehelin, 2006). Age per se has been shown not to be a good long-term predictor of functional autonomy, be it concerning ADL or IADL. Physical resources (especially mobility) turned out to be the best predictors for ADL, while IADL are best predicted by psychological resources such as memory (Perrig-Chiello et al., 2006). In the context of this thesis, it appears therefore that both cognitive and physical trainings might have a positive influence on functional autonomy; the physical trainings by way of improving mobility, and the cognitive training by improving memory.

*Frailty*

Frailty is one specific challenge of old age. The term refers to a decline in multiple systems combined with reduced physiological reserve. Symptoms include unintentional weight loss, muscle weakness, exhaustion and low physical activity. Frailty should not be confused with multimorbidity; even when patients with acute or chronic medical conditions are excluded, 20% of the over 80 year olds can be considered frail (Wilson, 2004). Frailty puts older people at a higher risk of functional limitations, impairments and finally institutionalization (Puts, Lips, Ribbe, & Deeg, 2005); furthermore, frail people are among the highest users of medical care (Wilson, 2004). However, it appears that frailty may be prevented or postponed; even more, it is a potentially reversible state. Several studies have shown that physical exercise is effective in decreasing functional decline in frail elderly people and reduces disability in activities of daily living (Gill, Baker, Gottschalk, Peduzzi, Allore, & Byers, 2002; Gill, Baker, Gottschalk, Peduzzi, Allore, & Van Ness, 2004).

From everything mentioned so far, it becomes clear that age-associated physiological changes are part of what is considered "normal" aging. However, there are great interindividual differences in the extent of these changes. Some older people remain almost unaffected to a very old age, whereas others become frail and dependent at a relatively early point. The interindividual variance is due to differences in individual resources. Resources will be discussed in more detail in a later section. It is also important to note that older people are not entirely at the mercy of fate - there is strong evidence that there are effective prevention and intervention strategies for many age-associated physiological changes.

However, age-associated physiological changes affect not only the body, but also the brain, and with the brain, cognition. The age-associated changes in the brain will be examined in more detail in the following section.

## 2.2 Changes in the aging brain

Changes in the aging brain are responsible for a great amount of cognitive difficulties that older people experience in everyday life, such as forgetfulness or trouble remembering names. To better understand what underlies the cognitive changes in old age, this section will provide a short overview over the changes in the aging brain.

*Neuronal loss and changes in neuronal architecture*

Neurons are postmitotic cells, meaning they have ceased to divide and will therefore not be replaced when they die. As a consequence, neuronal loss, when it occurs, is final and definite. Age-related neuronal loss begins at different times, depending on the brain area. Depending on the structure, abatement can start already in the early 20s, whereas other structures do not show any deterioration into old age. Even though some cell loss already occurs at a young age, Lezak (1995) states that "physiological [...] changes take place with increasing rapidity within the 50-65 age range". Thus, an older brain will consist of fewer neurons than a younger brain. Several studies have also confirmed a loss of brain volume with advancing age (Courchesne, Chisum, Townsend, Cowels, Covington, Egaas et al., 2000; Mueller, Moore, Kerr, Sexton, Camicioli, Howieson et al., 1998; Resnick, Pham, Kraut, Zonderman, & Davatzikos, 2003). Typically, as brain volume decreases, the volume of the cerebrospinal fluid increases (Resnick et al., 2003). There is some disagreement whether the rate of decrease of brain volume (and the correspondig increase in volume of the ventricles) remains stable in healthy aging or not (see Courchesne et al., 2000; Mueller et al., 1998 for opposing views on that issue). Not all areas of the brain show the same volume loss. Loss of gray matter with advancing age is most pronounced in orbital, inferior frontal, cingulate, insular, and inferior parietal areas. Mesial temporal lobes are also affected, but to a lesser degree, as are basal ganglia structures (caudate and lenticular nuclei, anterior thalamus). A majority of sudies have also reported a decrease in size of the hippocampus (Beason-Held & Horwitz, 2002). Taken all together, gray matter volume has been estimated to decrease by 2.4 $cm^3$ per year in healthy people older than 59 years old (Resnick et al., 2003). In addition to brain volume, brain weight also changes with age. It starts to decrease in people's thirties or forties and from then on declines progressively (Beason-Held & Horwitz, 2002).

Age-associated changes in the brain occur also on a deeper level, namely on the level of neuronal architecture. Several studies have found an age-related decline in dendritic extent (e.g. Nakamura 1985, as quoted in (Anderson & Rutledge, 1996). Additionally to dendritic decrease, a reduction of the number of neocortical synapses is also associated with advancing age – it occurs already from age twenty on (Masliah, Mallory, Hansen, DeTeresa, & Terry, 1993).

Another age-associated change in neuronal architecture concerns neuron size. It is not yet clear whether there is a reduction in neuron size or a decrement of bigger neurons. A decrease in the number of large neurons, accompanied by an increase in the number of small neurons has been observed in several newer studies (Beason-Held & Horwitz, 2002). However, this finding probably only applies to certain regions of the brain. A clear decrease in neuronal number (as opposed to a decrease in neuronal size) has been shown to exist e.g. in the hippocampus, thalamus, cerebellum, putamen, and several subcortical nuclei.

An increasing number of lesions in the white matter are also associated with aging. Estimates range from 54% (Boone, Miller, Lesser, Mehringer, Hill-Gutierrez, Goldberg, et al., 1992) to 95% (de Groot, de Leeuwe, Oudkerk, van Gijn, Hofman, Jolles, et al., 2000) of elderly displaying lesions in the white matter. Depending on extent and location, white matter lesions may have a detrimental effect on cognition (Boone et al., 1992); however, this topic is still highly controversial (Pantoni & Garcia, 1995).

A further change with advancing age is the increase of senile plaques and neurofibrillary tangles. An increase in tangle density is a normal part of healthy aging (Price & Morris, 1999). This cannot be said about plaques. Dani, Pitella, Boehme, Hori & Schneider (1997) state clearly that "NFT [neurofibrillary tangles] incidence, but not NP [neuritic plaques, i.e. senile plaques] incidence, correlated significantly with increasing age". A high incidence of senile plaques is associated with Alzheimer's Dementia, supporting the view that senile plaques are not part of healthy aging but an indicator for pathology.

*Changes in neurotransmitters and glucose metabolism*

Certain structural changes with advancing age cause age-correlated changes in the neurotransmitter systems, especially in the cholinergic and dopaminergic systems. It appears that after age 60, cells in the nucleus basalis of Meynert starts to atrophy, thus reducing the supply of acetylcholine. Furthermore, the receptors of the cholinergic systems appear also to be affected by age; one type of cholinergic receptor (muscarinic) has been found to decrease by 10-30% in the cerebral cortex and the striatum. The dopaminergic system is also affected by age-correlated changes. The neurons of the substantia nigra show a progressive decline after age 65 (Beason-Held & Horwitz, 2002). Noradrenergic neurons also decrease progressively from age 30-40 on. Adrenergic $\alpha_2$ receptors also decrease with age. In addition to all these changes in the neurotransmitter system mentioned above, old age also seems to be associated with a change in the reuptake of serotonin as well as with a reduction of receptor density (Beason-Held & Horwitz, 2002).

Further age-correlated changes in the brain can be seen on a metabolic level. Cerebral glucose metabolism tends to decrease with age (Moeller et al., 1996; Willis et al., 2002). However, not all brain areas are affected to the same degree. The glucose metabolism decreases mainly in the cingulate, frontal, temporal, insular and parietal cortex, whereas the cerebellum and visual cortex remain largely unaffected (Willis et al., 2002). Subcortical areas are in general less affected than cortical areas.

Up to this point, the majority of the discussed age-associated changes were not "illnesses", but simply part of so-called "healthy aging". However, old age is also a phase of life that is associated with an increased prevalence of many illnesses. These will be discussed in the next paragraph.

## 2.3 Age-associated illnesses and comorbidity

Due to the above-mentioned physical changes, illnesses and multimorbidity are a fact of old age. Typical age-associated chronic illnesses are atherosclerosis, cancer, diabetes, hypertension, heart disease, or osteoarthritis. 85% of people over 65 suffer from one or more chronic diseases (Bee & Bjorklund, 2004). Figure 1 shows the increase of a few select illnesses with age. However, even though morbidity increases in old age, there are risk factors involved (e.g. overweight, nutrition etc.) that may be modified and are thus partly responsible for the interindividual differences observed (Steinhagen-Thiessen & Borchelt, 1996).

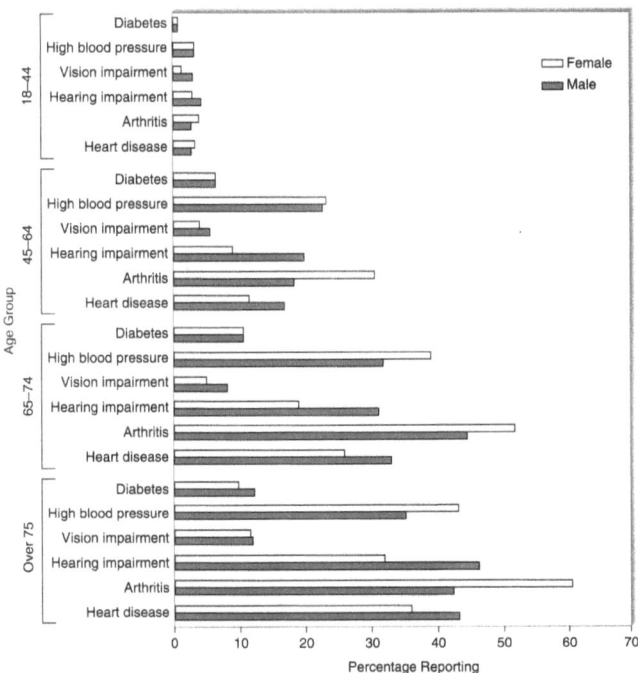

*Figure 1: Occurrence of chronic illnesses in different age groups in the United States (Bee & Bjorklund, 2004, p. 103)*

One age-associated illness that many older people fear is dementia, and especially (as it is the most frequent dementia) Alzheimer's dementia. This fear is understandable, as one percent of all 65-69 year olds suffer from a dementia, with the percentage rising exponentially with advancing age. Among the 90 year olds, already 35% are suffering from dementia. 60-70% of all dementias are of the Alzheimer type. Other common types are vascular dementia, Lewy-body dementia or frontotemporal dementia (Jahn, 2004). It is one of the challenges of the old to have to live with an ever-increasing probability of dementia as they grow older. The most frequent mental disorder (apart from dementia) in old age is depression, with a prevalence of 9% in the over 70 year olds. Data from the Berlin Aging Study (BASE) show that only few older depressed people are being treated with antipressants; in other words, this is a clear case of undermedication (Helmchen, Baltes, Geiselmann, Kanowski, Linden, Reischies, et al., 1996). This is a worrisome tendendy, especially in view of the fact that mental disorders are considered a causal factor for the loss of autonomy (Steinhagen-Thiessen & Borchelt, 1996).

One major concern in regard to age-associated illnesses is the simultaneous occurrence of several medical conditions (comorbidity). Comorbidity increases significantly with age in both men and women (Fortin, Bravo, Hudon, Vanasse, & Lapointe, 2005). 30% of people older than 70 years have five or more concurrent illnesses (Steinhagen-Thiessen & Borchelt, 1996). Associated with this is an increase in consumption of medical drugs with age. 75% of the participants of the Basle Interdiscplinary Study of Aging (IDA) were regularly taking one or several medications. Bloodpressure and heart medication are the front-runners amongst the regularly taken drugs (Perrig-Chiello, Staehelin, & Ehrsam, 1999, p. 85). The medical management of several coexisting illnesses is a challenge for both doctors and patients, as older people react differently to medication than younger people (due to changed pharmacokinetics), and multiple medications tend to interact. However, it is crucial to have an optimal medication management, as the quality of medication management has been shown to be significantly associated with the maintenance of functioning in old age (Steinhagen-Thiessen & Borchelt, 1996).

Clearly, in view of the age-associated changes mentioned so far, old age can be a challenging life stage. The term challenge, however, contains not only the element of difficulty, but also the element of opportunity. It is said that difficulties can make a person grow in different ways. According to different psychologists, difficult phases may for example lead to personality development. The next section will deal with the question if there is personality development in old age.

## 2.4 Personality development in old age

Numerous studies have found that personality traits are highly stable compared to other psychological constructs, such as e.g. moods (Roberts & Caspi, 2003). Personality dispositions like neuroticism, extraversion, and openness have been shown to be stable at least into people's seventies (Roberts & DelVecchio, 2000). It also appears that they become more stable with age. However, this does not mean that there are no changes in personality with aging. There are certainly interindividual differences, and different personality traits may also show different aging trajectories. Age gradients for extraversion and openness tend to be negative, while those for conscientiousness and agreeableness tend to be positive (Smith, 2003). As Roberts & Caspi put it, "personality consistency increases with age and yet may never reach a level high enough to indicate that personality traits stop changing. [...] Personality change can and does occur even into old age" (Roberts & Caspi, 2003, p. 185). They explain this statement with the fact that in every person's life, there are factors contributing to continuity and others contributing to change. Factors that contribute to continuity in personality include environmental influences (like one's socialization environment or social status), genetic influences, and person-environment transactions. Examples of such transactions are accommodative strategies (i.e. ajdustments in in goals or standards), which allow maintaining consistent self-views. Factors that contribute to change are responses to contingencies (i.e. responses to reinforcement or punishment), self-reflection, watching others (social learning) and listening to others (reacting to feedback we receive from other people about ourselves). It is the interplay of all these factors that leads to the fact that personality continuity does increase with age, but that there are also still changes in personality (Roberts & Caspi, 2003).

Closely related to personality development is the idea of developmental tasks associated with certain life stages. The probably most prominent of these theories was postulated by Erik Erikson. According to Erikson, personality development is achieved through a series of subsequent stages. Each of these stages is allotted to a certain age and is characterized by a psychosocial crisis or dilemma that needs to be resolved if personality development is not to be inhibited. However, people move on to the next stage even if they did not solve the previous stage's dilemma, carrying unresolved issues with them that may make the next dilemma all the more diffcult to solve. For Erikson, the last stage or dilemma of people's development is reached around age 60 or older, and is called „integrity versus despair". According to Erikson, this stage is usually precipitated when the person experiences a sense of mortality, be it through the death of a loved one, retirement, or another reason (Erikson, 1982). This experience of mortality leads the person to review and evaluate his/her life-career. The two extremes that can result from such a review are integrity or despair. Integrity denotes the acceptance of one's life career, a feeling of being embedded in family or society, and the acceptance of the finiteness of life. Despair on the other hand focusses on one's failures and missed opportunities, and the inalterability of the past. The solution of the psychosocial crisis is achieved by integrating both extremes; this is postulated to lead to wisdom. Erikson (1982) defines wisdom as a kind of "informed and detached concern with life itself in the face of death itself" (p. 61).

Other researchers have postulated different developmental tasks for old age. For McAdams, who sees the creation of a life story rather than the resolution of psychosocial crises as crucial for a person's identity, the developmental task of old age is the review, evaluation, reconciliation and acceptance of our life story (Sugarman, 2001, p. 101). Whereas as the early part of life is concerned with "story making", in old age the review of one's story becomes central. This view is compatible with Erikson's last developmental task insofar as an acceptance of one's life story may lead to integrity, while unhappiness with one's life story may lead to despair. As opposed to Erikson and McAdams, Newman & Newman (1995) have divided late adulthood into two stages, each with its own developmental task. Early late-adulthood encompasses the ages 60-75. The developmental tasks associated with this stage are promotion of intellectual vigor, redirection of energy toward new roles and activities, acceptance of one's life and development of a point of view about death. Late late-adulthood is from age 75 onwards, and contains the following developmental tasks: Coping with physical changes of ageing, development of a psychohistorical perspective, and "travel through uncharted terrain" (Newman & Newman, 1995). Common to all these theories is the view that there certainly is potential for development in old age just as in younger years. This is a challenge as well as an opportunity. Additionally, there is agreement that one important developmental task of old age is acceptance of one's life up to this point.

## 2.5 Age-associated changes in cognition

The age-associated changes mentioned in the previous section are extensive and concern different aspects of brain functioning and architecture. It can be expected that these changes may be interrelated with changes in cognition. However, the term cognition contains many different aspects, such as language, intelligence, memory, attention, speed, executive functions etc., which are differentially affected by aging. The focus will be on those areas of cognition that will be examined more closely in the empirical part of this thesis, namely memory, speed, and executive functions. To start, these terms will be situated. Following the definitions, an overview over some of the theories concerned with age-associated changes in cognition will be given. Finally, there will be a short summary of the empirical results concerned with age-associated changes in memory, speed and executive functions.

### *Situation of the terms memory, speed and executive functions*
*Memory*: According to the multi-store model of memory first postulated by Atkinson and Shiffrin (1968), memory involves sensory memory, longterm memory, and working memory. The sensory memory retains information in a fairly unprocessed form for a very short amount of time (a few hundred milliseconds). This information is stimulus-specific, i.e. depends on the manner of perception. In other words, we have a sensory memory for each sense (for visual, auditiv, haptic, and olfactory perception).

Longterm memory retains information for a theoretically unlimited amount of time. A distinction within long-term memory can be made between implicit and explicit memory. Explicit memory contents are conscious and can be verbalized. Explicit memory can be further subdivided into episodic and semantic memory. Episodic memory contents contain information about the time and place they were obtained, while semantic memory contents do not contain such information. In contrast to explicit memory, implicit memory contents cannot be verbalized. In implicit memory, previous experience influences present tasks without the person's conscious awareness (Schacter, 1987). This can be demostrated e.g. with priming experiments. Empirical evidence for the separation of implicit and explicit memory stems from studies with amnestic patients, in whom implicit memory is usually unaffected. Furthermore, several studies have shown that there are significant age-effects in explicit memory, while implicit memory appears to be age-resistant (Perrig & Perrig, 1993; Perrig & Perrig-Chiello, 1993).

The third main store in the Atkinson-Shiffrin model of memory is working memory. Working memory is used for temporarily storing and manipulating information. There are numerous theories about the exact structure and functioning of working memory. The three most widely acclaimed theories were postulated by Baddeley and Hitch (1974), Cowan (2005), and Ericsson and Kintsch (1995). According to Baddeley and Hitch, working memory contains the phonological loop, the visuo-spatial sketchpad, and the central executive. The central executive coordinates and controls the phonological loop and the visuo-spatial sketchpad. In 2000, Baddeley added a fourth component, the episodic buffer, which is capable of binding information from the other components and from long-term memory into a unitary representation (Baddeley, 2000). In contrast to Baddeley's model, Cowan (2005) considers working memory not as a system of its own but as part of long-term memory. Working memory consists of activated parts of long-term memory, some of which are within the focus of attention. Whereas there is no limit to the amount of information that can be activated in long-term memory, the focus of attention is capacity limited (to four chunks). Ericsson and Kintsch (1995), on the other hand, argued that in everyday life, we need a much bigger capacity than the 4-7 chunks that are usually postulated to be the capacity of working memory. Comprehending written information would for example not be possible with so few chunks. Ericsson and Kintsch therefore postulated that we actually store most of what we read in long-term memory. This information is linked by retrieval structures. Only very little information then needs to be stored in working memory, to serve as retrieval cue. This theory is usually referred to as "long-term working memory" theory. In this view, a person may have different working memory capacities depending on the situation. A chess master, for example, will have a great working memory capacity when plaing chess (as there are many chess moves stored in his long-term memory), whereas his capacity will normal in other areas of life (Ericsson & Kintsch, 1995).

*Speed:* The term speed can refer to speed of perception, motor speed, or speed of processing. Often, these three constructs are difficult to empirically separate (especially without the help of an electroencephalogram). When a person has to react to a certain stimulus by presssing a button, all three kinds of speed are involved. A person may be slow to see the stimulus, or the brain may be slow to process this input and connect it with the demand for motor movement, or the motor movement itself may be slow - of course, any combination of the mentioned options is also possible. Most of the time, therefore, speed is a conglomerate of the different factors mentioned above. According to Lehr (2003, p. 108), this conglomerate is usually termed psychomotor speed.

*Executive functions*

The term "executive functions" is normally used for a number of different mechanisms that enable flexible and intentional behavior and/or control other cognitive processes. The planning and controlling of actions, including inhibition and facilitation, are usually named as executive functions, as are the direction of attention and sometimes working memory. It becomes obvious that the mechanisms subsummed under this heading are extremely heterogeneous. Common to all is the fact that they appear to be located in the frontal lobe. The difficulty to define executive function is partly due to a lack of "process-behaviour correspondence", as Burgess (1997) has called the fact that there is no single particular behaviour that can be taken as an indicator of solely executive functioning (independently of any other functions). As the executive functions are mainly concerned with the control and coordination of other cognitive functions, they cannot be measured independently of the coordinated or controlled functions. At present, there is no satisfactory solution for this problem.

### *Theories of cognitive aging*

There are several theoretical approaches to explain age-related changes in memory and cognition, the most prominent ones focussing on a decline in processing speed, reduced processing resources, inhibitory deficits, impairment in executive control (Kester, Benjamin, Castel, & Craik, 2002), and reduced capacity.

The first approach states that a decrease in mental processing speed is responsible for the observed age-related decline in certain cognitive tasks (Salthouse, 1996). According to this theory, the slowing of processing speed results in an impairment due to two mechanisms, the limited time mechanism and the simultaneity mechanism. The limited time mechanism especially affects performance when there are external time limits for a task. In complex tasks, this can be problematic because the solution of most complex tasks relies on the results of several simpler operations. When time is limited and a person is slow, not all simple operations necessary to the solution of the complex task may be finished in time. Salthouse refers to this as the complexity effect, i.e. "the positive relation between task complexity and the magnitude of age differences in both speed and accuracy" (Salthouse, 1996, p. 404). The second important mechanism, the simultaneity mechanism, refers to the fact that the results of earlier processing efforts may already be lost again by the time that later processing is finished, by through decay or displacement.

This theory fits well with the finding that older people's performance is affected mainly in tasks requiring speed or high complexity. However, age-associated declines in free recall are more difficult to explain with this theory. Possibly the simultaneity mechanism could be involved, but in which way exactly is as yet unclear. In sum, even though the processing speed theory is an appealing approach to explain age-associated declines in cognition, there are still many open questions.

Another theoretical approach focusses on reduced processing resources to explain age-associated declines in cognition and especially memory (Craik & Byrd, 1982). This approach assumes that attention is necessary to do cognitive tasks, and that complex tasks require more attention than simple tasks. Older people have less attentional resources at their disposal, and thus may have problems with tasks that demand a great amount of resources. This theory could explain why older adults often have problems with deep and elaborate encoding of information, or with strategic search in retrieval, and why they they profit so much from cues and supportive contexts (Kester et al., 2002). Furthermore, it is supported by the fact that certain processes that are presumed to be automatic (such as implicit memory) are less affected by aging than other non-automatic processes (Perrig & Perrig-Chiello, 1993). However, one problem of the reduced processing resources approach is that its core concept, attentional resources, is only vaguely defined and difficult to distinguish from related concepts such as executive functions and working memory. Also, there are some (presumably) automatic processes such as spatial learning that do show age-related decrements (Kester et al., 2002). In sum, this theory is hard to test until its core concept is more clearly defined, and it cannot explain all findings.

Yet another approach postulates that an inhibitory deficit is causing age-associated cognitive decline (Hasher & Zacks, 1988; Hasher, Zacks, & Rahhal, 1999). In respect to memory, inhibition is important in at least three aspects. First of all, it restricts access to task relevant information. Second, it is responsible for deleting information that is no longer relevant from working memory. Last but not least, inappropriate responses are suppressed. Inhibitory problems could explain many of the memory problems older people' experience. In most cases, a lack of inhibition results in interference between different memory contents (old and new content, or appropriate and

inappropriate content, etc.). However, this approach cannot explain problems that are caused by a lack of activation rather than suppression (Kester et al., 2002).
The fourth approach is related to both the reduced processing resources and the inhibition approaches (Kester et al., 2002, p. 559). It postulates that older adults have an impairment in executive control. Therefore, automatic processes which do not require control would be expected to be unaffected by aging, whereas tasks demanding controlled processing would show age-associated decline. Even though this approach can account for many age-associated decrements, the problem is, just like with the reduced processing resources approach, the vague theoretical definition of "executive control". As long as it is not clear what differentiates this term from inhibition or attention or working memory, it is difficult to judge the usefulness of this theoretical approach.

None of the theories mentioned so far can (by itself) explain all the empirical findings concerned with aging and cognition. As of yet, it is still a matter of scientific debate how to best explain the observed findings. The most important empirical findings in regard to memory, speed and executive functions will be shortly summed up in the following section.

*Empirical evidence for age-associated decline in memory, speed, and executive functions*
*Age-associated changes in memory*: In memory there is a differential age-effect. Explicit memory clearly decreases with advancing age, while implicit memory remains largely unaffected. Sensory memory and short-term memory are not or only slightly affected by age, whereas long-term memory shows clear age-deficits (Davis & Bernstein, 1992). Working memory is one memory system that seems to particularly affected by aging processes. Its capacity is generally reduced in old people (Martin & Kliegel, 2005; Meier, 1999; Perrig, Meier, & Ruch-Monachon, 1999). However, it is difficult to say whether this may not be due to a decrease in executive processes (i.e. coordination of several processes) rather than storage capacity per se. Episodic memory also decreases with age, whereas semantic memory remains stable or may even increase (Kessler & Kalbe, 2000; for a digressing result, see Perrig et al., 1999). Furthermore, older adults seem to have „a particular deficit in memory that requires the binding of information to contextual elements" (Naveh-Benjamin, Guez, Kilb, & Reedy, 2004), which becomes apparent for instance in paired associate learning. Part of this result may be due to older people's reluctance to use strategies during encoding and retrieval (Touron & Hertzog, 2004). Here it becomes clear that it is difficult to consider just one cognitive function apart from all others – clearly, there is an interaction between memory, attention, and executive functions (strategy use is considered an executive function). Source memory, i.e. the memory of the context in which a certain information was first

encountered, shows also an age-associated decline (Martin & Kliegel, 2005). The results concerning aging effects in prospective memory, or the ability to remember to do something at a certain point of time in the future, are contradictory. However, there appear to be more and more studies that find an age-associated decline in this kind of memory, too (Martin & Kliegel, 2005).

*Age-associated declines in speed*:
As has been mentioned above, the term "speed" can refer to different constructs. Not all of these constructs are in the same way affected by aging. In reaction time tasks, it has been shown that the premotor component, i.e. the time between the appearance of a stimulus and the beginning of the movement, tends to get slower in older people. The motoric component, however, (i.e. the speed of the movement itself), does usually show less age-related decline (Lehr, 2003, p. 108). It has been debated whether the slowing of the premotor component is due to a slowing of information processing (as postulated by Cerella, 1985; 1990), or due to a slowing of peripheral processes (such as perception, see Strayer, Wickens, & Braune, 1987) However, a newer review has come to the preliminary conclusion that the decline in cognitive processing speed is not due to peripheral, sensomotor changes, but is most likely caused by a slowing of central information processing (Kessler & Kalbe, 2000).

*Age-associated decline in executive functions*
*Attention:* As in memory and intelligence, not all kinds of attention are affected by age to the same degree. Vigilance for instance remains unaffected. Selective and divided attention, however, show a clear decrease in old age. Older people are more easily distracted by unimportant information than younger people (Kessler & Kalbe, 2000).
*Planning, inhibition, flexibility*: Older people perform worse on the tower of London task (Davis & Bernstein, 1992) or the Wisconsin Card Sorting Task than younger people. Both these tasks demand planning ahead as well as the inhibition of non-optimal responses. The tendency to perseverate increases with age, and cognitive flexibility and the ability of abstract thinking are reduced (Kessler & Kalbe, 2000). As already mentioned, susceptibility to interference and distraction increases.
*Coordination of several tasks:* The ability to coordinate two simultaneous tasks shows a clear age-effect. Whereas the task that is in the focus of attention is only slightly affected, the secondary task shows clear decline (Meier, 1999).

In sum, most executive functions appear to be negatively affected by the aging process. However, one has to keep in mind that there are great interindividual differences, especially in an older population.

To sum up the age-associated changes in cognition relevant to this thesis, a decline with age is usually found in speed, episodic memory, working memory, and executive functions. In view of the losses associated with old age, the question arises whether they will negatively influence people's well-being. The next section will try to answer this question and give an overview over the construct of well-being and its determinating factors.

## 2.6 A special challenge: maintaining well-being in old age

**The concept of well-being**

Well-being is used quite loosely in everyday language to refer to a subjectively perceived positive state of being or in terms of the evaluation people make about the quality of their inner experience (Diener, 1984). This definition makes it difficult to distinguish well-being from related concepts such as quality of life or life satisfaction. Clearly, those terms need to be differentiated.

Quality of life refers mostly to a two-dimensional construct containing a subjective and an objective component (such as financial situation, housing, etc.) (Perrig-Chiello, 1997, p. 20; Stewart & King, 1991). The subjective component of quality of life can be termed well-being (Stewart & King, 1991). However, this does not elucidate what well-being actually is.

Well-being is usually considered to consist of several components. The probably most widely accepted view is that well-being contains the elements life satisfaction, positive affect and negative affect. However, positive/pleasant affect and negative/unpleasant affect form two independent factors (Bradburn & Caplovitz, 1965; Diener, Suh, Lucas, & Smith, 1999). It is possible for one person to experience high positive affect and very little negative affect, whereas a second person may experience high positive as well as high negative affect. This second person would probably be termed „highly emotional" rather than „happy" (Diener & Lucas, 1999). Therefore, although the three elements of well-being are related, they are assumed to be empirically separable (Diener & Lucas, 1999). Furthermore, well-being is usually considered to be a multidimensional construct which contains several components (Perrig-Chiello, 1997, p. 115). The three components most often mentioned are physical well-being, psychological well-being and social well-being. The extent to which these single components contribute to overall well-being may differ according to situation and person. A further distinction can be made between momentary and habitual well-being. This distinction is closely related to the question whether well-being is stable across time and situations. Could it be, for example, that there is an age-associated change in well-being? The next section will deal with this question in more detail.

**Well-being: stability or deterioration in old age?**

As was outlined in the first chapters of this thesis, old age is associated with many challenges and changes. Is age also associated with a decline in well-being?

As was stated in the definition, well-being is a construct that comprises different facets or components, namely life satisfaction, positive affect and negative affect. Research shows that these components are differentially affected by aging (Kunzmann, Little, & Smith, 2000). In regard to life satisfaction, several studies found that life satisfaction remained stable or increased with age (e.g.

Diener & Suh, 1998; Perrig-Chiello, 1997, p. 137). However, there are also a few studies that support a decline of life satisfaction in old age. It has for example been postulated that an overlay of cohort effects is responsible for covering up an actually existing decline in life satisfaction (Schilling, 2005). Data from the Berlin Aging Study also suggest that there may be a decline in life satisfaction (Smith et al., 2002). In regard to positive and negative affect, Smith and colleagues conclude that "decline is especially evident in the positive side of well-being: in aging satisfaction, life satisfaction, and positive affect. [...] In contrast, negative affect is characterized by average stability" (Smith, Fleeson, Geiselmann, Settersten, & Kunzmann, 1996, p. 726). Diener and Suh (1998) also confirmed that positive affect decreased from age 20 to 80, while negative affect remained unchanged. How could this decline in positive affect be explained? In a longitudinal study, Perrig-Chiello, Perrig & Staehelin (1999) found no decrement in psychological well-being, even though the amount of positive life experiences decreased with age. The finding that there are less positive life experiences in old age could partly explain the decline in positive affect with age. However, some researchers argue that it is the emotional intensity (whether positive or negative) that decreases with age, and not positive or negative affect per se (Diener, Sandvik, & Larsen, 1985). In the Berlin Aging Study (BASE), cross-sectional findings indicated that the experience of positive emotions may decrease from age 70 on, and become especially pronounced after age 80 (Smith et al., 2002). This finding confirms once again that there is a big difference between the so-called third age and the fourth age. It therefore appears that not only are different components of well-being differentially affected by aging, but also that there are differences according to the respective phase of aging. Then there is a further aspect: Just because there is a correlation between decline in the positive aspects of well-being and chronological age does not necessarily mean that it is age per se that causes the decline. Studies who took into account health in addition to well-being found that age-related variance in well-being can in fact be mainly attributed to health factors. In other words, it may not be chronological age per se that matters, but more the health problems often (but not always) associated with old age (Smith et al., 2002).

In sum, it appears that there is an age-associated decline in positive affect, whereas negative affect remains stable. The results concerning life satisfaction are less clear. In regard to well-being as a whole, most studies confirm stability (e.g. Perrig-Chiello, Perrig et al., 1999). Heady, Veenhoven and Wearing (1991) estimated the stability at 0.55-0.60 for two- to six-year intervals. While this may be regarded as fairly stable, the authors point out that this means nevertheless that "about a quarter of the population shift by over a standard deviation in these time periods" (Heady et al., 1991). This is once again confirmation of the high interindividual variance in old age.

In regard to the results mentioned so far, it also has to be mentioned that there is a sampling bias in most studies, as mainly moderately fit and healthy people are willing to participate in research projects. Elderly people who are institutionalized, in nursing homes or in hospitals are usually not represented in research samples. It is quite possible that the well-being of these subjects would differ markedly from their more or less healthy counterparts. Furthermore, there is also a positive selection bias in longitudinal studies, as the healthy elderly survive longer and are thus overrepresented in a study with several measuring points.

However, based on the results presented above it can be assumed that some aspects of well-being are stable, whereas others show age-associated decline. The fact that some aspects of well-being do change leads to the question of which factors can actually influence well-being. As the next section will show, this question is not that easy to answer.

**Well-being: top-down or bottom-up?**

In well-being research, one crucial question is which variables cause well-being and which are consequences of well-being (Heady et al., 1991). In other words, the direction of causation is often unclear. According to Diener (1984), bottom-up causation is when well-being is caused by particular variables. In other words, these variables are considered to be predictors of well-being. This builds on the idea that every person has basic needs, and that the fulfillment of these needs will cause positive well-being. In contrast, top-down theories of well-being postulate that well-being causes certain outcomes in particular variables (Diener, 1984); in other words, here the direction of influence is reversed, and well-being is the predictor for other variables.

Heady and colleagues (1991) tested the direction of influence/causality with structural equation modeling between well-being and six variables: Satisfaction with one's marriage, work, leisure, standard of living, friendship, and health (Heady et al., 1991). Results showed that there were different causations for different variables. Whereas marriage satisfaction and well-being mutually influenced each other, the variables work, leisure and standard of living showed top-down causation. The correlations between well-being and friendship and health were spurious (Heady et al., 1991). Furthermore, several other studies have shown that bottom-up processes such as age, income, education or situational circumstances can explain only about 15-20% of the variance of well-being (e.g. Argyle, 1999). These results would point more towards a top-down approach of well-being. However, there are also researchers who disagree with that opinion; for example, Blane, Higgs, Hyde, & Wiggins (2004) postulate that well-being in old age is determined mainly by „current contextual factors such as material circumstances and serious health problems". Analyses of data from the Berlin Aging study have shown that health was "a significant source" and "strong predictor" of well-being (Smith et al., 2002). Clearly, this issue is not resolved yet. Furthermore, it appears likely that there may not be a simple answer to the "top-down or bottom-up" question - the answer may differ according to the variable used. In the following section, several variables that have been postulated to be associated with well-being will be examined in more detail.

**Resources of well-being**

Resources are material, social or personal potentials of a person that s/he can use to deal with challenges or to make progress towards personal goals (Diener & Fujita, 1995; Jopp & Smith, 2006). The available resources differ from person to person. They include intrapersonal variables as varied as cognitive abilities, physical parameters, control beliefs and personality, as well as extrapersonal factors such as social contacts, social activities, aids, and financial standing. In other words, resources include everything a person has at his/her command to deal with different situations. Resources therefore determine not only whether a person is able to engage successfully in various activities, and which activities can be engaged in, but also how a person deals with success or failure in activities. In a bottom-up view of well-being, the extent and/or type of resources will determine a person's well-being. If one does not assume a strictly bottom-up approach, resources can be seen as correlates of well-being. Resources have been shown to be moderately strong predictors of well-being (Diener & Fujita, 1995). However, it is not just the total amount of resources that matters; when resources are relevant to a person's goal, they correlate more strongly with well-being than when they are not (Diener & Fujita, 1995). An ideal fit of situational demands and personal resources is therefore most beneficial for well-being.

There are many different ways in which resources can be grouped. One possibility is to distinguish between physical, psychological and social resources (Perrig-Chiello, 1997). Another possibility, which is used in this thesis, is a categorization according to whether resources are intra- or extrapersonal. In second step, the intrapersonal category is then further divided into cognitive, physical and personality-related resources, while the extrapersonal category contains social resources as well as aids (e.g. hearing aids), socioeconomical status and environmental factors. Extrapersonal resources such as money and material possessions have been shown to be less relevant to people's well-being than intrapersonal resources (Diener & Fujita, 1995). Therefore, the focus will from now on be on intrapersonal resources. A selection of intrapersonal resources, which are considered especially important for well-being, will now be examined in more detail.

*Physical resources: Health*

When talking about health, one has to distinguish between objective and subjective health. Often, and this is true especially for old age, there is only a weak or no significant correlation between the two measures (Perrig & Perrig-Chiello, 1999). It has been shown in several studies that the subjective perception of health is a better predictor for well-being than objective health measures (Diener et al., 1999; Kozma, Stones, & McNeil, 1991, p. 73). Subjectively perceived health complaints and well-being are highly correlated (Perrig & Perrig-Chiello, 1999). Analyses of the data collected in the Berlin Aging Study have also shown that "functional health constructs and subjective health were significant sources of SWB", with subjective health being the strongest predictor of well-being overall (Smith et al., 2002, p. 726). In this study, health accounted for 20% of of the variance in life satisfaction, 14% in negative affect, and 13% in positive affect. Subjective health appeared to have a strong influence on life satisfaction, while functional health seemed to matter more for positive affect (Smith et al., 2002). It is important to mention that the perception of one's health may be strongly influenced by control beliefs. These will be discussed in more detail in a section of their own.

*Personality-related resources*

Personality is one of the strongest predictors or correlates of well-being (Diener et al., 1999; Ruch-Monachon, Perrig-Chiello, & Staehelin, 1999). It has also been shown that personality traits are highly stable over the years (Ruch-Monachon et al., 1999), which is something personality has in common with well-being. Heritability studies with twins have shown that there is a genetic predisposition to higher or lower well-being (Tellegen, Lykken, Bouchard, Wilcox, Segal, & Rich, 1988) - one could call it a temperamental disposition. The link between personality and well-being is supported by the fact that well-being tends to be quite consistent not only over time, but also across different situations. However, certain situations can influence well-being. As Diener and colleagues put it, "personality predisposes people to certain affective reactions, but [...] current events also influence one's current levels of SWB" (subjective well-being) (Diener et al., 1999). With that in mind, some personality-related resources will now be examined in more detail - for a more complete coverage of the topic, please consult Diener et al., 1999.

**Extraversion and neuroticism**: The personality traits most often mentioned as being related to well-being are extraversion and neuroticism, with extraversion being moderately correlated with positive affect and neuroticism being strongly correlated with negative affect (Diener & Lucas, 1999). Between 4 and 10% of the variance of well-being can be explained by neuroticism and extraversion (Kozma et al., 1991). The influence of personality could contribute to the stability of the well-being construct, as personality is highly stable compared to other psychological variables (Roberts & Caspi, 2003). As Smith and colleagues put it, "in part, stability is a function of enduring personality characteristics" (Smith et al., 2002). However, there are other personality-related resources apart from extraversion and neuroticism that may contribute to well-being. One of the most prominent one is control beliefs.

**Control beliefs**: As Abeles, Gift and Ory (1994) state, "Sense of control and quality of life for older people are intimately interrelated. Sense of control is a pivotal contributor to wide variety of behaviors and to both mental and physical well-being, which are essential elements of quality of life" (p. 297). The construct "locus of control" (which is a more exact term for sense of control) denotes a system of expectations regarding who or what is responsible for outcomes in the subject's life (Wallhagen, Strawbridge, Kaplan, & Cohen, 1994). Persons with an internal locus of control believe that they have control over what is happening to them; they feel in charge. In contrast, people with an external locus of control believe that their life events are determined by external forces and are thus beyond their control. Externality and internality are not extremes of the same dimension (Molinari & Niederehe, 1984-85) but independent. External locus of control is often divided into two subscales, powerful others and chance. A belief in powerful others implies that others have control over events in one's life. A high score on the chance subscale implies a belief that everything in life is due to fate or coincidence and that there is nobody who can have any effect on outcomes. An internal locus of control is usually associated with positive well-being and life satisfaction, whereas external locus of control has been linked to depression. As Perrig-Chiello summarizes it, the more personal control a person thinks s/he has, the better the outcome for well-being (Perrig-Chiello, 1997, p. 74). Several researchers have postulated that people become more external with age, due to an actual loss of control experienced in daily life (e.g. Wolinsky, Wyrwich, Babu, Kroenke, & Tierney, 2003). However, others have postulated that older people are more internal than younger people (Rhee & Gatz, 1993). The discrepancy is mainly between studies using unidimensional scales. There is a clearer consensus between studies using multidimensional scales (meaning studies differentiating between internal and external control, or even between internal, powerful others and chance subscales). These studies generally agree that internal control beliefs remain stable or decrease slightly, while external control beliefs increase (Lachman, 1991). A newer study by Perrig-Chiello (2000) confirms this statement: In an Inter-Disciplinary study on Ageing (IDA), longitudinal results yielded that scores on the powerful others and chance subscales increased significantly with age, whereas internal health related control beliefs remained stable and thus appear to be age-resistant. An important finding of this study was that there were gender effects. Women showed lower internality and powerful others scores than men (Perrig-Chiello, 1999, 2000). Similar findings were reported by Gatz and Karel (1993), Ross and Mirowsky (2002), or Wallhagen and colleagues (1994). Education may also have an influence on control beliefs; persons with lower education levels have been reported to have higher powerful others scores than people with higher education levels (Perrig-Chiello, 1999). It is possible that people with higher education are more critical towards authorities and therefore less inclined to accept that ohers may have power over them. Apart from education, marital status has also been shown to be associated with certain patterns in control beliefs. Singles and divorcees tend to have lower internality scores than married people (Perrig-Chiello, 1999).

**Resilience**: Resilience can be defined as a potentially protective personality trait (Leppert, Gunzelmann, Schumacher, Strauss, & Brähler, 2005), which enables a person to withstand adverse circumstances and deal effectively with challenges. Or, as Kahn & Juster define it, "the ability to recover quickly and completely from [...] misfortunes and challenges" (Kahn & Juster, 2002). In old age, this includes being able to adapt to losses and functional decline (Leppert et al., 2005; Staudinger, Freund, Linden, & Maas, 1996a). A Study by Leppert et al. (2005) found a significant positive association between resilience and life satisfaction. Resilience proved to be a better predictor for subjective complaints than age or gender. Very resilient elderly people are characterized by more positive affect, optimism, and lower neuroticism than their less resilient counterparts (Staudinger, Freund, Linden, & Maas, 1996b, p. 346).

*Cognitive resources:*
Clearly, cognition is an important resource for everyday functioning. Many people are very afraid of losing their intellectual faculties in old age, of experiencing deterioration in memory and of becoming confused. As was mentioned in the section "age-associated changes in cognition", however, only some aspects of cognition decline with age, whereas others remain stable. Cognitive functioning has been shown to be positively related to life satisfaction and positive affect in the elderly, independent of educational levels (Jones, Rapport, Hanks, Lichtenberg, & Telmet, 2003). As with the resource "health", it may be useful to distinguish between subjectively perceived and actual cognitive functioning. It has for example been shown that the subjective perception of one's memory performance is a better predictor of well-being than objective memory performance (Perrig-Chiello, 1997, p. 180).

It has therefore been shown several times that the individual's *perceptions* of his or her resources is crucial for well-being. This implies a strong and also somewhat active involvement of the individual in the maintenance of well-being. The next section will further elaborate on this topic.

**Regulation of well-being**

As has been shown above, there are many variables that contribute differentially to well-being. It would be wrong, however, to assume that the simple presence or absence of resources alone determines a person's well-being. The maintenance of well-being in old age is a permanent process of regulation, in which the person concerned can play an active role. The extent and nature of a person's active involvement differs depending on the applied regulation theory. Three of these theories will now be examined in more detail.

According to the first theory, the hedonic treadmill or adaptation theory of well-being (Brickman & Campbell, 1971), there is nothing much a person can do do affect longterm well-being. It postulated that, similarly to processes of sensoric adaptation, an adaptation occurs when people experience positive or negative life events. Due to this adaptation, the hedonic level quickly returns to neutrality (Diener, Lucas, & Scollon, 2006). Some parts of the hedonic treadmill model have received empirical support (see Frederick & Loewenstein, 1999, for a review). However, lately several adjustments to the original model have been postulated. Diener and colleagues (2006) name five important points of revision: First of all, research has shown that people's hedonic set points are not neutral but in most cases positive. Second, there is great interindividual variance in set points. Third, different aspects of well-being (e.g. positive affect and negative affect) may have different set points. Fourth, it is now believed that a longterm change in well-being is possible. Last but not least, it is stated that there are individual differences in adaptation. All these points are supported by empirical data (for details, see Diener et al., 2006). Even though the original hedonic treadmill could not be upheld in its original form, its adapted version helps explain why many changes in people's lives have only a small influence on long-term well-being. At the same time, it also suggests that "interventions to increase happiness can be effective" (Diener et al., 2006).

Another model of regulation was postulated by Baltes and Baltes (1990). It is called the model of selective optimization and control (SOC), and is based on a framework of propositions. These propositions are: (1) There are differences between normal and pathological aging; (2) There is much heterogeneity in aging; (3) There is much latent reserve; (4) There is an aging loss near limits of reserve; (5) Knowledge-based pragmatics and technology can offset age-related decline in cognitive mechanics; (6) with aging the balance between gains and losses becomes less positive; (7) the self remains resilient in old age (Baltes & Baltes, 1990, pp. 7-19). Based on these propositions, the authors describe a general process of adaptation. The first element of this process is selection,

„which refers to an increasing restriction of one's life world to fewer domains of functioning because of an aging loss in the range of adaptive potential. It is the adaptive task of the person [...] to concentrate on those domains that are of high priority [...]. Although selection connotes a reduction in the number of high-efficacy domains, it can also involve new or transformed domains and goals of life" (Baltes & Baltes, 1990, p. 21).

An example of this would be an aging athlete who notices that he cannot keep up a high level of performance in both tennis and skiing. He could therefore decide to concentrate on tennis alone. The second element, optimization, refers to behavior that maximizes the results in the selected domains (qualitatively and quantitatively). To return to our example, the above mentioned athlete will probably have to train more to keep up with his old performance level, and he may decide to improve his technique rather than his stamina, as this promises greater success. The final element, compensation, is a consequence of the restricted plasticity in old age. When functioning in a certain area cannot reach a certain level anymore, people can try to compensate with the help of technology (e.g. with a hearing aid for hearing problems, or in the above mentioned example with a better racquet) or with psychological compensatory efforts (mnemonic techniques for memory problems, etc.). The authors believe that selective optimization with compensation is a promising strategy for successful aging (Baltes & Baltes, 1990), which contains the maintenance of positive well-being. The SOC model has received a lot of attention and has also received empirical support. For example, Jopp and Smith were able to show that SOC strategies had a lasting influence on well-being, this especially in resource-poor individuals (Jopp & Smith, 2006). However, the SOC model has also been criticized for focussing too much on limitations instead of on growth potentials and resources (Lehr, 2003).

Other regulation models have focused more on the possibility that well-being in old age may be strongly mediated by subjective perception and attribution processes. It has for example been postulated that older people lower their aspirations. This could explain why worsening external factors like deteriorating health do not lead to a decrease in well-being. Brandtstädter's model of assimilative and accommodative coping is an example for that viewpoint. It gives a possible explanation for the phenomenon that people who live under adverse circumstances nevertheless often report high well-being. According to Brandtstädter's model, a balance between goal pursuit and goal adjustment makes it possible to maintain a positive perspective over the lifespan (Brandtstädter, 2002). The term assimilation refers to a person's attempt to alter a situation or the course of personal development so that it matches personal goals. In other words, the person sticks to his or her goals and increases his/her effort to reach them. In the case of the elderly, this may involve an increased time investment (more practice) or compensatory activities (such as e.g. focussing more on strategy than strength in sports) (Brandtstädter, 2002). However, assimilation places high demands on a person's resources. At a certain point, it may not be possible any more to compensate for an age-associated decline by increased time investment or compensation. At that point, acommodation comes into play. Accommodation denotes the adjustment of aims and goals to situational constraints. This may involve disengaging from a goal, readjusting one's ambitions or changing comparison perspective. It has been shown that older people who emphasize accommodation report greater satisfaction with their aging (Brandtstädter, 2002). It therefore appears that the adjustment of goals to what is actually feasible may play an important role in the maintenance of well-being in old age.

Both the SOC model and the model of assimilative and accommodative coping show that old people are not helpless and passive pawns of the aging process - rather, they play an active role in determining their own well-being.

# 3 How to Deal with the Challenges of Well-Being and Cognition in Old Age: Effects of Intervention Studies

As has been shown above, certain areas of cognition show a clear decline with advancing age. It would therefore be of great interest to find methods to revert this decline or to compensate for it. Usually, as people age, they develop their own strategies to compensate for certain losses (e.g. by writing down appointments etc.). Apart from compensating, another option is to adjust one's expectations (as has been discussed in the section on regulation of well-being). However, there is is also the possibility of selectively training certain functions that are usually affected by age. It is this last option that shall be examined in more detail for its efficacy in the following section. This thesis focusses on physical and cognitive training in old age; other kinds of trainings (such as self-awareness or relaxation etc.) will not be covered. Furthermore, we will restrict the literature review to training studies that were concerned with effects on cognition and well-being.

## 3.1 Physical training effects on cognition in old age

Studies from as early as 1927 showed that very brief, high intensity exercise may lead to a facilitation of cognitive processes if assessed during the exercise session (for a review see Tomporowski & Ellis, 1986). The facilitation was greatest at moderate levels of intensity. Later studies examined whether there was also a facilitation effect right after exercise. The results of these studies differed widely. Some found a facilitation effect 2-5 minutes after exercise, which turned into impairment after 10 minutes (Davey, 1973; Gupta, Sharma, & Jaspal, 1974), whereas others found no effect (Flynn, 1972; Gutin & DiGennaro, 1968b) or even an impairment of cognitive function (Gutin & DiGennaro, 1968a). All these studies did not, however, answer the question whether there is a persistent, long-term effect of exercise on cognition. This is a crucial question in terms of everyday benefits of exercise for the elderly.

Many cross-sectional studies measuring reaction times as indicators of long-term effects of exercise found that people who exercise regularly have significantly lower reaction times than their age-matched sedentary peers (these were not intervention studies). Even more impressively, it has been shown that very fit older participants may be as fast as people who are several decades younger (for a review, see Stones & Kozma, 1996). Intervention studies were less equivocal in their support of the benefits of physical training on cognition (for an overview of intervention studies, see Table 1). Some reported improvements (e.g. Dustman, Ruhling, Russell, Shearer, Bonekat, Shigeoka et al., 1984; Kramer, Hahn, Cohen, Banich, McAuley, Harrison, et al., 1999) while others did not find any positive change in cognition (e.g. Blumenthal, Babyak, Moore, Craighead, Herman, Khatri, et al., 1991; Hill, Storandt, & Malley, 1993). In the studies reporting improvements, benefits were mainly found for measures involving speed (Dustman et al., 1984; Rikli & Edwards, 1991), memory span (Hassmen, Ceci, & Backman, 1992; Williams & Lord, 1997), or free recall and recognition (Perrig-Chiello, Perrig, Ehrsam, Staehelin, & Krings, 1998).

Table 1: Overview of studies concerned with the effect of physical training on cognition

| authors | year | n | age | type of training | no-training control group | length of intervention | results on cognition |
|---|---|---|---|---|---|---|---|
| Blumenthal et al., 1991 | 1991 | 101 | 60-83 | aerobic (bicycle, walking, jogging) vs yoga | X | 4 - 14 months, 3times/week, 45min | no group differences in memory, psychomotor speed and Stroop |
| Dustman et al., 1984 | 1984 | 43 | 55-70 | aerobic (walking, running) vs strength | X | 4 months, 3 times/week, 60min | improvement of aerobic group only in Digit Symbol, simple reaction time, Stroop |
| Emery & Gatz, 1990 | 1990 | 48 | 61-86 | aerobic exercise vs social activity vs waiting list | X | 12 weeks, 3times/week, 25min aerobic exercise (60min overall) | no improvement in digit symbol test, digit span or writing speed |
| Hassmen et al., 1992 | 1992 | 32 (all women) | 55-75 | walking | X | 3 months, >3times/week, 20min | no effect on simple reaction time, but improvement on digit span |
| Hawkins, Kramer, & Capaldi, 1992 | 1992 | 36 | 63-82 | swimming | X | 10 weeks, 3times/week, 45min | improvement in time-sharing and dual task for exercise group compared to controls |
| Hill et al., 1993 | 1993 | 87 (exp) 34 (ctrl) | 60-73 | walking, running (individually prescribed) | X | 12 months, 3-5 times/week 50min | no effects on long-term memory (WMS), psychomotor speed and working memory |
| Kramer et al., 1999 | 1999 | 124 | 60-75 | walking vs. stetching and toning | - | 6 month (no further information) | Improvement in task switching, response-compatibility, and stopping test (all considered to measure executive function) |
| Madden, Blumenthal, Allen, & Emery, 1989 | 1989 | 85 | 60-83 | aerobic vs yoga | X | 16 weeks, 3times/week, 45min | no exercise-related improvement in reaction-time tests of attention and memory retrieval |
| Moul, Goldman, & Warren, 1995 | 1995 | 30 | 65-72 | walking vs weight training vs placebo (flexibility training) | - | 16 weeks, 5times/week, 30-60min | improvement in Ross Imformation Processing Assessment (RIPA) of aerobic group |
| Okumiya, Matsubayashi, Wada, Kimura, Doi, & Ozawa, 1996 | 1996 | 42 | 75-87 | aerobic (walking, game playing) | X | 6 months, 2times/week, 50min | no change in Mini Mental State or Dementia Scale (HDSR) |
| Perri & Templer, 1985 | 1985 | 23 (exp) 19 (ctrl) | 60-79 | walking, jogging | X | 14 weeks, 3times/week, 30min aerobic act. | no improvement in short-term memory |

35

*Table 2 (continued)*

| | | | | | | |
|---|---|---|---|---|---|---|
| Perrig-Chiello et al., 1998 | 1998 | 46 | 65-95 | resistance training | X | 8 weeks, once/week, eight exercises | sign pre-posttest changes in recognition and free recall (free recall still sign. after one year) |
| Rikli & Edwards, 1991 | 1991 | 21 (exp) 13 (ctr) | 57-85 | low impact aerobics | X | 3 years, 3times/week, 60min (20min aerobic exercise) | simple and chioce reaction time improved (participants all female) |
| Williams & Lord, 1997 | 1997 | 94 (exp) 93 (ctrl) | >60 | aerobic exercises and strengthening | X | 42 weeks, twice/week, 60min aerobic and flexibility | reaction time and memory span improved (participants all female) |

Opinions differ as to whether the exercise has to be aerobic (i.e. leading eventually to an improvement in cardiovascular functioning) to be beneficial for cognition. Kramer and colleagues (1999), for example, found an exercise effect only for aerobic, but not for anaerobic (stretching and toning) training. Dustman and colleagues (1984) found greater effects for aerobic training than non-aerobic training (but with both groups outperforming a no-training control group). Evidence for the effectiveness of a non-aerobic training stems from a resistance training program by Perrig-Chiello and colleagues (1998), which yielded significant positive effects on free recall and recognition. The evidence is therefore mixed and complicated by the fact that the definitions of "aerobic" differ and most researchers do not denote whether their program should be considered aerobic or anaerobic. However, Tomporowski and Ellis (1986) state that "[u]nder normal conditions, almost all exercise involves a combination of anaerobic and aerobic energy production". Therefore, the distinction may be mainly academic and not matter for most types of exercise performed by the elderly in their normal environment.

Meta-analyses were conducted to assess the effect size across studies. Etnier, Salazar, Landers, Petruzzello, Han and Nowell (1997) came to the conclusion that even though effect sizes were largest when a correlational design was used (effect size = 0.53), chronic exercise "does have a small positive impact on cognitive functioning" (effect size = 0.33). Another meta-analysis of aerobic fitness intervention studies conducted between 1966 and 2001, by Colcombe and Kramer (2003), found a significant effect of aerobic fitness training. The performance of the participants increased on average by 0.5 standard deviations (effect size: 0.48). Executive processes benefited most from the fitness interventions. Furthermore, exercise interventions that combined aerobic components with strength and flexibility training were more effective than aerobic exercise alone. Last but not least, it was found that the exercise duration is another important factor. The effects on cognition were greatest for trainings that took longer than 30 minutes per session.

In summary, meta-analyses and reviews yield strong evidence that physical exercise is indeed beneficial for certain aspects of cognition, such as executive functions, speed and memory.

The hypothesized reasons for these effects lie in the physiological changes exacted in the brain by physical training. Animal studies have shown that metabolic and neurochemical functions improved with increased aerobic fitness (Black, Isaacs, Anderson, Alcantara, & Greenough, 1990; Neeper, Gomez-Pinilla, Choi, & Cotman, 1995) and may even cause permanent structural changes in the brain (Black et al., 1990). Some studies with humans have also demonstrated the benefits of aerobic exercise for the brain. Colcombe, Erickson, Raz, Webb, Cohen, McAuley, and colleagues (2003) found that aerobic fitness plays a moderating role in age-related tissue density decline. Neurotransmitter levels are also affected by exercise. Several studies have found increases in norepinephrine (Mitchell, Flynn, Goldfarb, Ben-Ezra, & Copman, 1990), serotonin (Barchas & Freedman, 1963), as well as in endorphins (Bortz, Angwin, Mefford, Boarder, Noyce, & Barchas, 1981). Exercise furthermore causes an increase in cerebral blood flow (Hellström, Fischer-Colbrie, Wahlgren, & Jogestrand, 1996; Ide & Secher, 2000). All these factors likely contribute to the positive effect of exercise on cognition. However, there may also be psychological and social factors involved. Physical training may provide participants with heightened self-efficacy. The term self-efficacy refers to „the belief that one possesses the necessary skills of complete a task as well as the confidence that the task can actually be completed with the desired outcome" (Craft, 2005). When people experience that they are able to complete a physical training program, and when they perceive the positive effect thereof, this may strengthen their belief that they are capable human beings. Support for this theory is found, amongst others, in a study by Craft (2005). She found increased levels of self-efficacy in the exercise group after nine weeks of exercise, whereas self-efficacy in the control group did not increase. Increased self-efficacy may then lead to increased confidence, which decreases stress in test situations. This alone can already lead to an improvement in cognitive tests. An additional factor that may explain part of the physical exercise effects on cognition is that most trainings take part in groups. This may increase the amount of social interaction that the elderly participants take part in. Social interaction is cognitively stimulating, thus possibly contributing to the observed effects on cognition. Most likely, it is an interplay of physical, psychological and social factors that cause the positive effects of exercise on cognition.

## 3.2 Cognitive training effects on cognition in old age

There is a wealth of studies concerned with improving cognitive functions. As this thesis focusses on older people, the review will be limited to studies with an older population. To gain an overview, cognitive trainings with older people can be divided into certain categories (Knopf, 2001). A first category contains training programs that stem from the "testing the limits"-approach (Kliegl & Baltes, 1991; Kliegl, Smith, & Baltes, 1989). In these programs, a sample of elderly is typically taught a method with which to solve a specific problem. Then they practise this method extensively. It has been shown that elderly who have been trained this way can outperform much younger adults who did not receive any training. This category of trainings tries to fully exhaust the cognitive reserve capacity and plasticity of older people. In these studies it has been clearly shown that intensive cognitive training of a specific method leads to an improved performance in the practised tasks. However, the practical benefit of such a program for everyday life is highly doubtful. First of all, the time investment for practice is very high considering that the gain/improvement applies only to one specific task. Second, these tasks were often laboratory tasks and thus not transferable to everyday life. In conclusion, these studies were very useful for showing that older persons' cognition can be improved quite drastically; however, they were not designed to be a help for everyday tasks in participants' lives.

A second category of cognitive training programs, which is closely related to the first, teaches the participants mnemonic strategies, like the method of loci, imagery or elaboration. However, in contrast to the first category, these training programs do not aim to exhaust the reserve capacity; therefore, there is no period of intense practice comparable to the one in the testing the limits approach. Most training programs belong to this category (Knopf, 2001). Many studies show that mnemonic techniques are effective in improving performance in comparison to control conditions (see Ball, Berch, Helmers, Jobe, Leveck, Marsiske, et al., 2002; Verhaeghen, Marcoen, & Goossens, 1992). However, a general problem with mnemonic strategies like the method of loci is that participants do not continue to use them after instruction (see e.g. Scogin & Bienias, 1988, who conducted a three-year follow-up of a memory skills program). Furthermore, the learned techniques are very task-specific and the benefits do not usually generalize to other tasks (Verhaeghen et al., 1992). One exception to this can be found in a study by Noice, Noice, Perrig-Chiello and Perrig (1999), in which a special and augmented form of elaboration was taught to older adults. In this study, participants were instructed in professional acting techniques. These techniques included analyzing the characters' aims and goals, and putting oneself in that character's position and speaking the lines with those goals in mind. Other techniques were improvization, subtextual exploration and Alexander technique. Participants then practiced a scene and performed it in front of others. The training took four weeks. The results showed that the acting training led to a significant improvement in immediate recall, delayed recall and recognition of word lists. Therefore, in this study a transfer effect was actually found, which is extremely rare with mnemonic techniques. Maybe this was was due to the combination of different approaches, some of which demanded emotional involvement. However, in this study as in other studies concerned with mnemonic techniques, the question remains whether there are any long-term benefits; furthermore, it has to be stressed that usually mnemonics do not generalize to other tasks.

The first two categories of cognitive training focussed on imparting very specific tools for specific situations. The third category, on the other hand, aims to optimize memory in a more general way that could potentially benefit a broad range of everyday situations. Stigsdotter and Bäckman (1989), for example, added a training of attentional functions and a relaxation training to the traditional mnemonics approach. The group who received this multifactorial training showed a significant improvement in the memory of concrete words. However, the positive effects did not generalize to other memory-related tasks such as digit span or visual retention. The observed improvement for concrete words was greater in the multifactorial than the mnemonics-only group, and was stable for six months after posttest. In a second follow-up three and a half years later (Neely Stigsdotter & Bäckman, 1993), the level of performance was unchanged, indicating to the authors that "memory training may result in long-term effects for older adults in tasks that are congruent with the training activity". However, results from this study as well as from a later one by the same authors (Stigsdotter Neely & Bäckman, 1995) show that there is only a very restricted range of generalizability to tasks other than the trained ones, despite the multifactorial approach.

A different, but also multifactorial approach was pursued by Wolters, Bemelmans, Spinhoven, Theunissen & van der Does (1996). These authors used a program that focussed on teaching general knowledge about memory functioning instead of teaching specific mnemonics. Mnemonics were only touched on cursorily as an illustration of strategies that can be used in certain instances. Participation in the training resulted in an improvement in word-list tasks and in a face-name-association task. This improvement was unchanged in a follow-up test two months later. A similar approach was used in a later study by Mohs, Ashman, Jantzen, Albert, Brandt, Gordon, et al. (1998), who also found an improvement in the learning of word lists that remained stable for two months after posttest (but had disappeared at the six month follow-up). However, none of the other measures used in the study showed any improvement, i.e. that again there was no transfer effect on tasks other than list learning.

A fourth category focusses on improving memory or other cognitive functions by cognitive restructuring, or in other words, improving the motivational aspects. One way to achieve better motivation is to offer a reward for good performance. Hill, Storandt, and Simeone, for example, offered their participants a free lottery ticket for every correctly remembered word (Hill, Storandt, & Simeone, 1990). However, the incentive failed to improve performance in a skills training group (in comparison to a skills training group that did not receive an incentive). Yesavage and colleagues (1982, 1990) hypothesized that not a lack a motivation was the problem, but rather that anxiety impairs the performance of elderly people. Therefore, he set out to test whether teaching the participants relaxation techniques might improve memory performance. However, in both his studies relaxation failed to have a positive influence on memory performance (Yesavage, Rose, & Spiegel, 1982; Yesavage, Sheikh, Friedman, & Tanke, 1990). Another approach is to try and enhance memory function by encouraging positive beliefs about memory in old age. Caprio-Prevette & Fry (1996) compared such a cognitive restructuring program to a program teaching traditional memory techniques. The cognitive restructuring showed a greater effect not only at posttest, but also after an interval of nine weeks. Becca Levy took a similar approach. Levy believes that negative self-stereotyping can have a detrimental influence on memory performance in older people (Levy, 1996). She was able to show that an activation of positive stereotypes about aging without the participants' awareness improved their memory performance, while an activation of negative stereotypes led to a decline in memory performance (Levy, 1996). This finding was supported by other studies concerned with the effect of stereotype activation on memory performance (e.g. Hess, Hinson, & Statham, 2004). Other researchers confirmed that stereotype threat (i.e. that a relevant stereotype is made salient in a performance situation, like for example aging stereotypes in a memory test) may have a detrimental effect on memory (Rahhal, Colcombe, & Hasher, 2001; Schmader & Johns, 2003). Effects were also found on other measures such as walking speed (Bargh, Chen, & Burrows, 1996; Hausdorff, Levy, & Wei, 1999). Opinions differ whether the presence of stereotype threat is enough, or whether a stereotype activation (as conducted by Levy) is necessary to create the effect. However, most authors agree that it is important that the stereotype activation happens without the participants' awareness (this independently of whether the stereotypes were presented subliminally or not) (Hess et al., 2004; Stein, Blanchard-Fields, & Hertzog, 2002). In summary, the activation of stereotypes and/or the reduction of stereotype threat appear promising candidates to improve memory in the elderly.

Finally, there are quite a few trainings that do not fit into just one of the above mentioned categories, as they combine different approaches. An example of such a training program is the SIMA program (Rupprecht et al., 1993). In addition to classical mnemonics, this program also contained a competence training for the management of everyday situations as well as a psychomotor training. This training yielded „highly significant specific improvements of the trained functions" (Oswald, Rupprecht, Gunzelmann, & Tritt, 1996). One problem with programs that combine different approaches, however, is that it is almost impossible to determine which part of it is actually responsible for the observed effects. Furthermore, no transfer effects on non-trained functions were reported. Another training that does not quite fit into any of the above mentioned categories is a working memory training conducted by Klingberg, Forssberg and Westerberg (2002). These authors used an adaptive training task of working memory on children with ADHD (attention deficit hyperactivity disorder) and later young adults without ADHD. Not only did the training improve working memory (WM) performance, it also improved performance on two non-trained tasks, namely a visuo-spatial working memory task and a non-verbal complex reasoning task. The authors conclude that „[t]hese results demonstrate that performance on WM tasks can be significantly improved by training, and that the training effect also generalizes to nontrained tasks requiring WM" (Klingberg et al., 2002). Since then, these findings have been confirmed by other studies (Buschkuehl, 2007). Seeing as all more complex cognitive and memory tasks (apart from pure span tasks) require working memory, this approach appears very promising for future training programs.

It is very difficult to compare the different types of trainings, as the trainings themselves, the participants, the duration of programs etc. vary widely. However, there are two meta-analyses concerned with memory training with older participants that may shed some light on the issue. One meta-analysis is from 1997 and included 27 studies (Floyd & Scogin, 1997), ten of which had also been included the earlier meta-analysis by Verhaegen et al. (1992). The main difference between the two meta-analyses is that Floyd & Scogin assessed *subjective* memory functioning, whereas Verhaeghen & colleagues assessed *objective* memory functioning. Even though there was an improvement in subjective memory measures ($d_{++} = .19$), this was less than the improvement observed in objective memory measures by Verhaeghen and colleagues ($d_{++} = .73$). As this thesis focusses on objective memory measures, the results of Floyd & Scogin's analysis will not be discussed in more detail.

The meta-analysis by Verhaeghen, Marcoen and Goossens from 1992 included 33 studies with participants aged 60 and older. This analysis yielded that pre-posttest improvement was significantly larger in treatment groups ($d_{++}=.73$) than in control ($d_{++}=.37$) or placebo groups ($d_{++}=.38$) (see Table 2). Verhaeghen et al. also computed the effect sizes as function of the type of mnemonic taught (Table 3). Results show the name-face and organization mnemonics were the most effective. Furthermore, the age of the participants and the duration of the training session had a negative affect on improvement scores (Verhaeghen et al., 1992). However, one of the weak points of this meta-analysis is that effect sizes were calculated only for target measures and not for measures that could be taken as indicators of a generalization of the training to non-trained functions (which was one of the aims of the training created as part of this thesis). Furthermore, the meta-analysis focussed only on mnemonics and did not include other approaches such as working memory training.

*Table 2: Effect sizes of memory training in comparison to controls or placebo*

| Measure | k | $d_+$ |
|---|---|---|
| Total sample | | |
| Control | 10 | .38 |
| Placebo | 8 | .37 |
| Memory Training | 49 | .73 |
| Studies including a control condition | | |
| Control | 10 | .38 |
| Memory Training | 14 | .68 |

Note: Adapted from Verhaeghen et al. 1992. k= number of effect sizes; $d_+$ = mean weighted effect size.

*Table 3: Effect sizes of different kinds of mnemonics*

| Mnemonic | k | $d_+$ |
|---|---|---|
| Method of loci | 12 | .80 |
| Name-face | 14 | .83 |
| Pegword | 2 | .62 |
| Imagery (paired associates) | 1 | .14 |
| Organization | 2 | .85 |
| Total (single) | 31 | .81 |

Note: Adapted from Verhaeghen et al. 1992. k= number of effect sizes; $d_+$ = mean weighted effect size.

As has already been discussed earlier, one problem of mnemonics is that they do not generalize to other tasks. Therefore, even though their effectiveness has been proved in the meta-analysis mentioned above, they are not suitable if one wants to achieve generalized effects (see Table 4). In consideration of everything said so far, a program that combines different approaches, including stereotype activation and working memory training, appears the most promising if one aims to achieve cognitive training effects that transfer to tasks other than the ones that were trained. This conclusion was taken into consideration in the design of the cognitive training used in the ExTrA study.

*Table 4: Different types of cognitive training and their respective effects*

| type of training | example of authors | effect on trained functions | effect on non-trained functions | long-term effects |
|---|---|---|---|---|
| "testing the limits" - approach | Kliegl & Baltes 1991 | yes | no | not assessed |
| mnemonics | Scogin & Bienias 1988 | yes | no | no |
| elaboration & acting | Noice, Noice, Perrig-Chiello & Perrig 1999 | yes | yes | not assessed |
| multifactorial (mnemonics, attention, relaxation) | Stigsdotter & Bäckman, 1989; Rupprecht et al. 1993 | yes | no | yes |
| cognitive restructuring | Hill, Storandt & Simeone, 1990; Yesavage, 1990 | - | no effect on memory | not assessed |
| positive stereotype activation | Levy 1996 | - | positive effect on memory performance | not assessed |
| working memory training | Klingberg et al. 2002 | yes | yes | not assessed |

## 3.3 Comparison of physical and cognitive training effects on cognition

Having examined the training effects of physical and cognitive training in turn, of course the question appears which of the two types of training would be superior in improving cognitive function. So far, only one study exist that is concerned with this question and directly compared physical and cognitive training in respect to cognitive function. In this study by Fabre, Chamari, Mucci, Masse-Biron, and Préfaut (2002), an aerobic training group was compared to a mental training, a combination of aerobic and mental training and a control group. Mental training sessions took place once a week for 90 minutes, over a time period of two months. The mental training focussed mainly on stimulating different functions such as attention, sight, hearing, association and imagination. Participants practiced certain mnemonics to better remember social security and bank account numbers. The test used to assess memory at pre- and posttest was the Wechsler Memory Scale (WMS). Results showed that the combined training (aerobic plus mental) was more effective than either aerobic or mental training alone in improving memory function. There was no difference between aerobic and mental training; both improved memory function to the same degree (one-way analysis of variance of the mean difference between pre- and posttest; Fabre et al., 2002). The authors give neither effect sizes nor enough information so that effect sizes could be computed. In short, this study concludes that aerobic training and mental training "could induce the same degree of improvement in cognitive function" (Fabre et al., 2002). A combination of the two trainings led to significantly greater improvements than each training alone. However, one single study (which employed quite a novel cognitive training) is not enough to determine whether physical and cognitive training really do have similar effects on cognition. More information can be gained by comparing the effect sizes of different meta-analyses. Verhaeghen et al. (1992) observed an effect size of .73 in objective memory measures for cognitive training (in this case, only mnemonics). In comparison, the meta-analyses concerned with physical training yielded effect sizes between .33 (Etnier et al., 1997) and .48 (Colcombe & Kramer, 2003). From these numbers it appears that cognitive training is more effective. However, there is a caveat: Most of the studies with mnemonics used test procedures that were very close to the trained tasks (whereas this was of course impossible for the physical trainings). It is well known that mnemonics do not yield generalized effects. Therefore, even though the mnemonics were highly effective in the test situation, their effectiveness does not apply to other cognitive tasks, and their everyday usefulness is limited. As there is no meta-analysis that assesses the mean effect size of other types of cognitive training and their effectiveness on different tasks, the effect size of Verhaegen et al. cannot be generalized to all kinds of cognitive tasks.

## 3.4 Physical exercise effects on well-being

*Studies with depressed participants*

One hint that physical exercise may have a beneficial effect on well-being comes from studies with depressed persons. Positive and negative affect are, as already mentioned, an element of well-being (Bradburn & Caplovitz, 1965). Depression can therefore be considered a pathological state of well-being. Depression as pathology and the healthy range of well-being will be treated separately here. The short review of literature is limited to studies with an elderly sample.

Depression is characterized by „depressed/gloomy" mood, loss of interest, joylessness and reduced drive (World Health Organization, 2007). Traditionally, depression is treated with psychotropic drugs and/or psychotherapy. However, there has also been a great interest in alternative treatment options such as physical exercise.

A literature search yielded six published studies that have examined the more long-term effect of exercise on depression in over 50 year olds. McNeil, LeBlanc and Joyner (1991) conducted a training study with elderly people (mean age 72.5) in which an experimenter-accompanied walking group was compared to a social contact group and a normal control group without increased social contact. The time of social contact was the same in both experimental groups. Results showed that both groups with social contact were equally effective in reducing psychological symptoms of depression. However, only the exercise group managed to reduce the somatic symptoms of depression. It thus appears that even though social contact seems to be important in combating depression, it cannot account for all the effects. Furthermore, this study showed that physical exercise could be an effective antidepressant in older people.

The question remained whether a different type of exercise might be just as effective in the treatment of depression. Singh, Clements and Fiatarone (1997) conducted a study in which 17 clinically depressed elderly persons (all older than 60) participated in a progressive resistance training for 10 weeks. Aften ten weeks, participants in the resistance exercise condition showed significantly reduced depression scores in comparison to controls. Therefore it seems that walking as well as progressive resistance training may be an effective antidepressant.

Seeing the positive performance of aerobic training in the treatment of depression, the question arises whether its effects could be comparable in magnitude to the effects of medication. To this purpose, (Babyak *et al.*, 2000) conducted a study which compared aerobic training to treatment with a selective serotonin-reuptake inhibitor (SSRI, in this case sertraline) and to a combination of aerobic exercise and sertraline. All participants had been diagnosed with major depression and were at least 50 years old. After four months of treatment all three groups had significantly improved; the level of improvement was very similar in all three groups. Six months after the end of treatment, however, the authors state that „remitted subjects in the exercise group had significantly lower relapse rates than subjects in the medication [or combined] group". An older study by Blumenthal, Babyak, Moore, Craighead, Herman, Khatri et al. (1999) with very similar design (same groups) had yielded much the same effects, i.e. all groups showed reductions in depression scores. Furthermore, the magnitude of these reductions was comparable to the levels achieved by using sertraline in other trials. According to these two studies, then, aerobic exercise appears to be as effective as medication in the treatment of depression, if not more effective in the long run.

An extensive literature search yielded three review articles concerned with the effect of physical activity on depression, one by North et al. (1990), Lawlor & Hopker (2001), and one by Phillips et al. (2003). However, as none of these reviews focussed on older participants, they will not be discussed any further, other than to say that the newest of them, the review by Phillips et al. (2003), concluded that the few randomized studies conducted with clinically depressed patients all found aerobic exercise to be as effective or more effective than other interventions (including medication and psychotherapy).

Popular explanations for the positive effect of exercise on depression include the self-efficacy approach (see e.g. Craft, 2005), the time-out or distraction hypothesis (Nolen-Hoeksema, 1991), the amine hypothesis (Ransford, 1982), or the endorphin hypothesis (Drevets & Raichle, 1992). However, as the focus of this thesis lies not on depression but on well-being in a non-pathologcial sample, these explanation models will not be discussed any further. For the moment, let it suffice to say that exercise does appear to have a beneficial effect on depression. Seeing the positive effect of exercise in the treatment of depression, the question arises whether exercise may also be helpful in increasing wellbeing in a non-pathological sample.

*Studies with non-depressed participants*

Several studies as well as reviews and metaanalyses concerned with that question were conducted in the past years. Most of the intervention studies conducted found a positive effect of exercise on various variables related to well-being. Norris, Carrol and Cochrane, for example, compared an aerobic training group to an anaerobic and a control group (Norris, Carroll, & Cochrane, 1990). The aerobic group showed larger changes in measures of wellbeing and stress than the anaerobic group; both experimental groups showed greater changes than the control group. A study by McAuley et al. (2000) compared aerobic exercise to a toning/stretching group and found no difference between the two groups. Both groups showed an improvement in well-being, which indicated in the opinion of McAuley et al. that the aerobic aspect did not matter. A similar result comes from a study by King, Taylor & Haskell (1993), who compared endurance trainings of differing intensities. All experimental groups showed a reduction in anxiety and perceived stress compared to a control group; however, there was no difference between the different intensity-groups. A study by Perrig-Chiello, Perrig, Ehrsam, Staehelin & Krings (1998) which assessed the effects of resistance training on well-being yielded more differentiated results. While the sense of well-being did not change in the elderly participants, there was a significant increase in self-forgetfulness, which indicated that the participants were less anxious. Therefore, while this study found no direct effect on well-being, there was nevertheless an effect on another variable which might indirectly influence well-being. All studies mentioned up to now are summarized in Table 5.

*Table 5: Overview of intervention studies concerned with the effect of physical training on well-being*

| authors | year | groups | result |
|---|---|---|---|
| McAuley et al. | 2005 | Aerobic exercise vs. stretching/toning, 6 months, 3x per week | Linear increase in positive wellbeing over first 4 months, with subsequent plateau for the last 2 months |
| McAuley et al. | 2000 | Aerobic exercise vs. stretching/toning | Both groups improvement in wellbeing => aerobic aspect does not matter |
| Perrig-Chiello et al. | 1998 | resistance training vs control, 8 weeks, 1x per week eight resistance exercises | No change in sense of well-being, but increase in self-forgetfulness in resistance training group |
| King et al. | 1993 | Endurance high intensity group, endurance high and low intensity home, controls; 1 year, 3x60min | Experimental groups greater reduction in anxiety and and perceived stress; no difference between three experimental groups |
| Norris et al. | 1990 | Aerobic, anaerobic, control, 10 wks training, 3x45min | Aerobic > anaerobic, aerobic + anaerobic > controls |

Apart from the studies mentioned up to now, a number of reviews and meta-analyses have also been published that were concerned with the question whether exercise was beneficial for well-being in the elderly. For example, Spirduso and Cronin (2001) state the following:

*„In large sample correlational studies and prospective longitudinal studies, researchers consistently report that measures of physical function in old adults are related to feelings of well-being, and that old adults who are physically active also report higher levels of well-being and physical function, but the results of randomized intervention studies of aerobic and/or resistive strength training do not always support this relationship."*

A second, a bit older review by McAuley & Rudolph (1995) also finds an association between physical exercise and psychological well-being in the majority of the 38 studies examined. Furthermore, the authors reported a positive association between length of exercise program and more positive results (for a detailed table of all studies used and their outcomes please consult McAuley & Rudolph, 1995). The studies included were concerned with either exercise programs (mainly aerobic exercise), acute bouts of exercise or physical activity assessed by subjects' retrospective recall (i.e. in this last case there was no intervention). However, one problem is that the authors included studies with participants older than 45, so that in the end there was a mean age of 56.7 years. The findings of such a review may not generalize to a population of 80 year olds.

A meta-analysis by Arent, Landers & Etnier (2000) applied more strict selection criteria in terms of age, aiming for ages older than 65. This meta-analysis included 32 studies that "investigated the effects of physical activity or exercise on some construct of mood in older adults" (Arent et al., 2000) and came to the conclusion that „chronic exercise is associated with improved mood in the elderly", with lower intensity more beneficial than high intensity training programs (which is contrary to McAuley & Rudolph's findings), whereas a long duration of the intervention did not seem to matter. In this study, mood improvements were found for all types of exercise (overall effect size of 0.24 for treatment versus comparison effects), particularly for resistance training.

The newest meta-analysis is from 2005, by Netz, Wu, Becker & Tenenbaum. It aimed to inlude all English-language studies from before 2004 that examined the effect of exercise or physical activity interventions on adults older than 55 and provided sufficient statistical information. 36 studies were included in the final analysis, the oldest stemming from 1982, yielding quite differentiated results. First of all, physical activity was found to have a positive effect on well-being, with aerobic activity and moderate intensity levels being most beneficial. The findings concerning exercise duration were inconclusive, but seemed to point in the direction that longer exercise duration was less beneficial for several types of well-being (Netz et al., 2005).

In summary, there is substantial evidence that exercise has a positive effect on well-being in a non-pathological sample. The two meta-analyses yield contradictory evidence as to whether aerobic or non-aerobic training such as resistance training is more beneficial. Similarly, it is not clear yet which duration of exercise would be best. However, exercise is clearly a valid way to improve well-being in older adults.

## 3.5 Cognitive training effects on well-being

In comparison to the wealth of studies concerned with physical training effects on well-being, there are only few studies concerned with cognitive training effects on the same. However, as the most frequently voiced complaints of the elderly relate to memory and cognition it would make sense that a subjectively experienced decline or improvement in this area could have an influence on well-being. Scogin, Storandt, & Lott (1985) examined the effectiveness of a memory-skills training on memory complaints, memory performance, and symptoms of depression (as indicator of well-being). They found a significant impact of the training on memory performance; however, despite this improvement, memory complaints and symptoms of depression remained unaffected. This result implies that neither memory complaints and actual memory performance nor memory complaints and depression are systematically related. Wolters, Theunissen, Bemelmans, van der Does and Spinhoven (1996) also conducted a short memory training program including a pre-post assessment of well-being. There was a significant increase in well-being from pre- to posttest, however, as this increase happenend in the training as well in the control group, it can be interpreted as a test-retest effect. A meta-analysis which analyzed the effects of memory training on subjective memory functioning and mental health of older adults (Floyd & Scogin, 1997) comes to a similar result. Even though the trainings led to improved subjective memory functioning, there was no difference to the control groups regarding mental health measures. These results could indicate that a benefit in cognitive performance obtained in a training study may not necessarily cause an increase in well-being. It is difficult to reconcile these findings with studies that identified cognitive functioning as predictor of well-being. For example, Jones, Rapport, Hanks, Lichtenberg & Telmet (2003) found cognitive functioning to be predictive of life satisfaction and positive affect, but not of negative affect. However, physical health and perceived health were stronger predictors than was cognitive status. The fact that there was no change in negative affect may also serve to explain why Scogin et al. and Floyd & Scogin, who used depression as sole indicator of well-being, did not find an association. It seems to be the case that negative affect is not a sufficient indicator of well-being, and that more encompassing measures of well-being yield better results. In conclusion, it appears that cognitive functioning can have an influence on well-being, albeit not a very strong one, and only on certain aspects of well-being (presence of positive affect, and not absence of negative affect).

In sum, even though there is some evidence that cognitive functioning is associated with well-being, so far there are not enough intervention studies to come to a conclusion as to whether cognitive training may have a positive effect on well-being. So far, intervention studies have found no effects that were unique to the experimental condition. In view of this, one could assume that physical training would be a more effective means to improve well-being than cognitive training. The next section will deal with the comparative effectiveness of physical and cognitive training in regard to well-being.

## 3.6 *Comparison of physical and cognitive training effects on well-being*

The easiest way to assess whether physical or cognitive training has a greater effect on well-being would be by directly comparing them in the same study. However, despite an extensive search of literature, only one study was found that directly compared the effects of physical and mental training. Furthermore the dependent variable was quality of life and not well-being. Nevertheless, the results of this study will quickly be delineated here. Fabre, Massé-Biron, Chamari, Varray, Mucci and Prefaut (1999) compared an aerobic training to a mental training, a combination of both and a control group. The mental training focussed mainly on memory improvement by teaching association strategies. The dependent variable in respect to quality of life was the subjective quality of life profile (SQLP). Results of the study yielded that the trainings that contained physical training showed an improvement in the domain of „functional life" which contains questions pertaining to fitness, tiredness etc. In comparison, the mental training intervention did not lead to a change in functional life. The degree of satisfaction pertaining to the experienced change was also greater in the physical training groups than in the mental training group. In sum, this study indicates that physical exercise is more effective in influencing well-being than cognitive training.

Furthermore, in view of the fact that the meta-analysis of Netz et al. found a weighted mean-change effect size of 0.24 for physical activity, whereas Floyd & Scogin conclude that "depression and mental health measures [...] were not responsive to memory training programs" (and a calculation of the effect sizes in their paper reveals an average effect size of -0.03 for mental health measures and 0.014 for depression), it has to be stated that at present (and until further evidence can be collected) physical exercise appears to be better suited to improve well-being than cognitive training. More studies on cognitive training and its effect on well-being are needed, especially ones that assess "well-being" per se instead of depression or mental health. Until then, it remains unclear if cognitive training (namely memory training) has a beneficial effect on well-being at all.

Up to this point, the reader has been given an overview over the state of the art regarding physical and cognitive training with the elderly and its effectiveness on cognition and well-being. These findings served as basis for the development of the cognitive intervention program in the ExTrA study. The rationale for the development of this intervention will be explained in more detail in the following section.

## 3.7 Rationale for the psychological intervention in ExTrA

Up to this point, it has been shown that aging is usually associated with changes in body, brain, and cognition. In some older people, certain aspects of well-being (such as posititive affect) are also affected. However, it has also been shown that there are great interindividual and intraindividual differences in the age-associated changes. Furthermore, elderly people are not helpless pawns in the hands of fate; they are active contributors and agents in regard to their development in old age. As has been elaborated in the section on physical and cognitive intervention studies, training is one possibility to influence cognition and well-being in old age. Many studies have been conducted on the effect of either cognitive or physical training on cognition and/or well-being; however, few studies have directly compared the two different types of training and in addition assessed well-being as well as cognitive variables. The ExTra study aims to fill this gap.

The intervention used in the ExTrA study is based on a resource- and activity model. The activity approach assumes that those people will be content in old age who are active and who accomplish things (Lehr, 2003). Several studies have shown a positive influence of activity on well-being and contentment; one of the earliest probably being the study by Maddox (1963), who found a relationship between activity and „morale" in a sample of 182 elderly subjects. Another study found that continuing volunteer work and occupational work were positive predictors of well-being for the elderly (Holahan, Holahan, & Wonacott, 2001). Results such as these lend support to the activity theory. However, the activity theory is not without its flaws. A frequently criticized point is that the activity model lacks any information about the type, diversity and demand level of the activities. Furthermore, it doesn't take into account individual differences, such as a person's resources. Therefore, in this model, the general idea of the activity theory, namely that staying active is crucial for „successful aging", is combined with a resource approach. Using Perrig-Chiello's resource model of well-being (1997, p. 146) as a basis, resources are considered predictors of well-being (see also "resources of well-being", section 2.6). However, for the use in this study, the resources were grouped according to different criteria than those used by Perrig-Chiello, into intrapersonal and extrapersonal resources. The intrapersonal resources can be further divided into cognitive, physical, and personality-related resources (see Figure 2). When an activity is undertaken, the task difficulty determines the outcome in interaction with the person's resources. If the task is too easy, people get easily bored and distracted; if the task is too difficult, people get frustrated and de-motivated. An optimal fit between a person's ability (which is determined by resources) and task difficulty will lead to positive well-being and continued engagement in the task. The heightened well-being from this first activity is then itself a resource for the next activity undertaken.

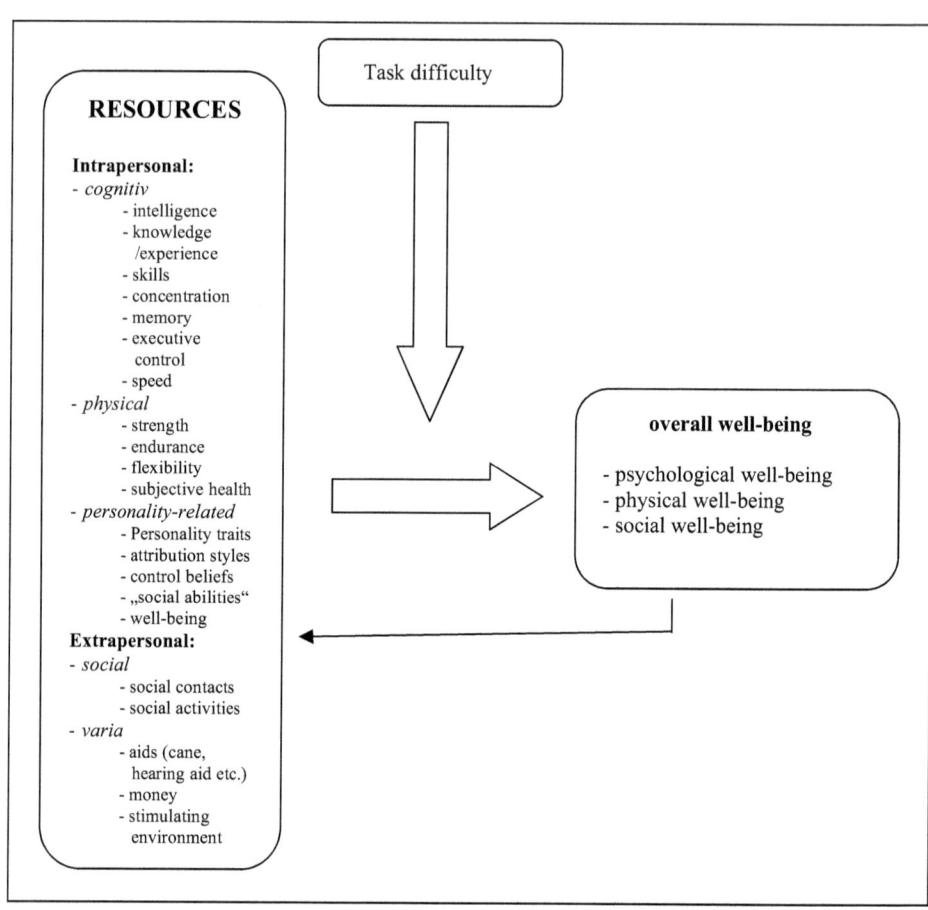

*Figure 2: Resource model of well-being (based on Perrig-Chiello, 1997)*

In the ExTra study, participants were supplied with activity that presented an optimal fit between task difficulty and each person's individual resources (the tasks adapted to each person's performance level). Two groups participated in physical activity (either eccentric training or resistance exercises) and one group in a cognitive training. In all groups, the demand level was adapted to the participants' performance level. However, in addition to the task difficulty, certain cognitive processes may also influence the success of an intervention. As was shown in the literature review above, stereotypes about aging may influence older people's performance in cognitive and physical tasks. Therefore, the cognitive training also included the activation of positive attitudes about aging.

The model proposed here postulates that cognitive as well as physical activity will have specific as well as non-specific effects. Physical activity is assumed to increase the trained physical parameters (specific effects), as well as non-trained physical and cognitive parameters (unspecific intervention effects). Similarly, it is expected that performance in trained cognitive tasks will improve, but that there will also be unspecific intervention effects on non-trained tasks as well as on parameters such as well-being. **Fehler! Verweisquelle konnte nicht gefunden werden.** illustrates the intervention model for the cognitive training group. The ExTrA study as a whole and the different trainings will be described in more detail in the following section.

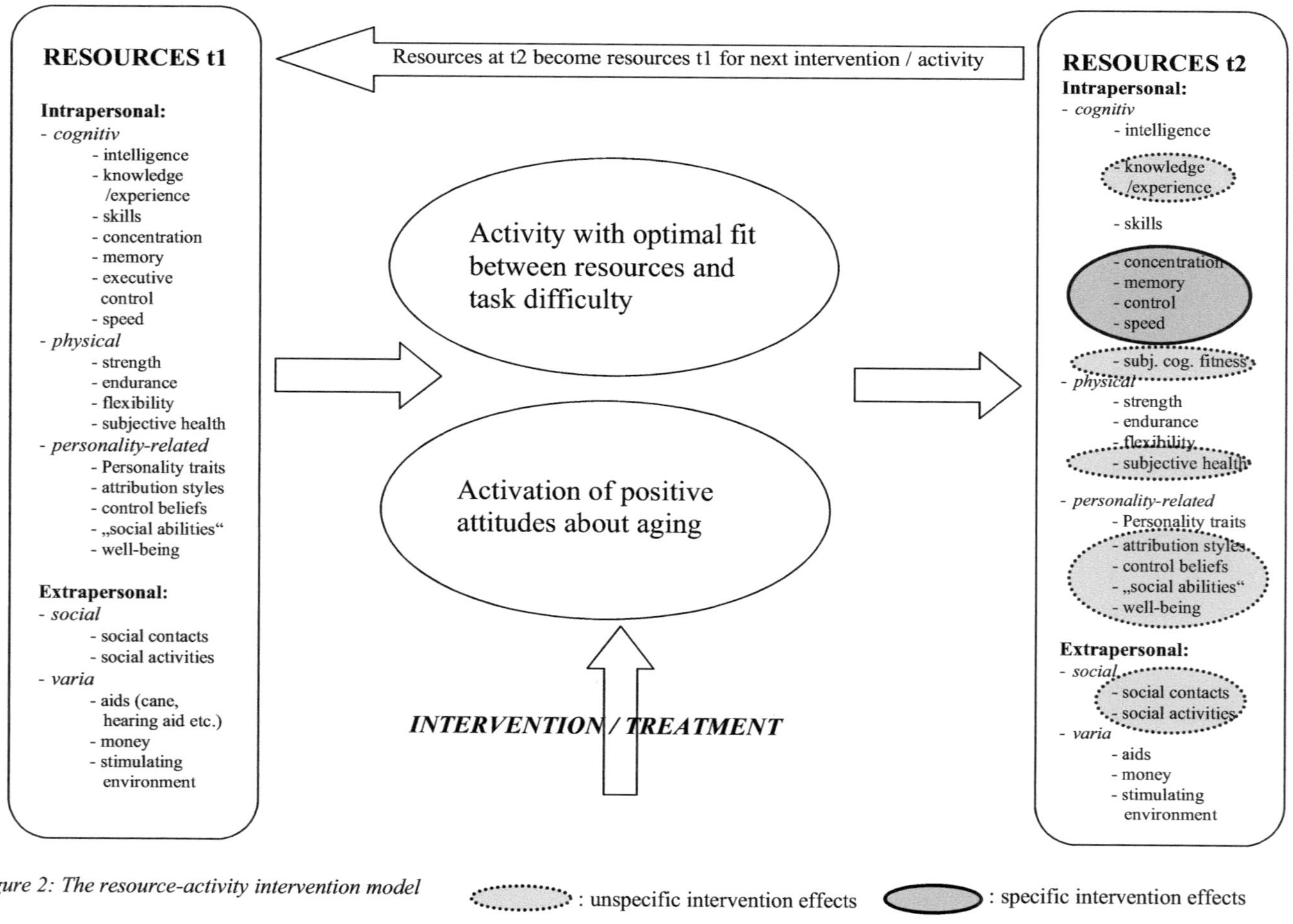

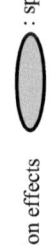

Figure 2: *The resource-activity intervention model*

# 4 Method

## 4.1 Design

After a health check and familiarization with test procedures, participants took part in physical and psychological testing (pre-test). After that, they trained for three months in one of three training groups, either eccentric strength training, conventional strength training, or cognitive training. Training sessions took place twice per week and took about 45 minutes. After three months of training, participants were tested again with the same tests as at pre-test. One year after post-test, a follow-up testing took place for participants who had completed the training (Figure 3).

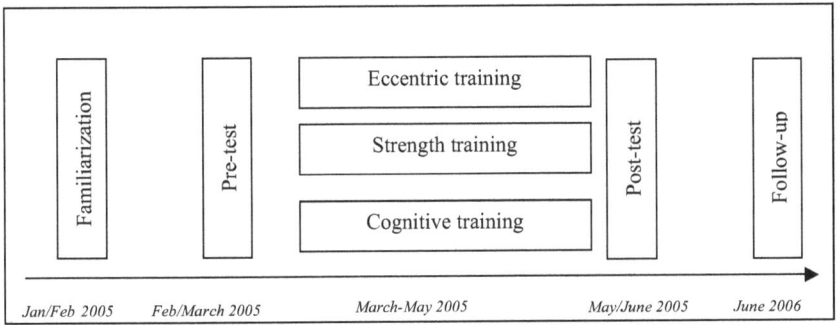

*Figure 3: Overview of the structure of the ExTrA study*

## 4.2 Sample

The initially planned sample size was 48 persons overall (16 per group). The number 48 was determined by the fact that it would have been impossible to train more than 16 people in each of the three training groups due to temporal, monetary and personnel constraints. Participants had to be at least 80 years old and in good health. As the response rate after sending 1000 letters to participants of the senior's university of Berne had been very low, it was decided to recruit participants in a different way. For this, personal visit were made to senior sports groups, where the study was introduced and participants were personally invited to an information meeting. Furthermore, the inclusion criteria were softened to include people 75 years and older. At the information meetings (meetings were held several times), participants were informed in detail about the study, inclusion criteria and associated requirements and risks. At the end of the meeting, they were given detailed information in writing, a sign up slip and a sheet on which they had to confirm that they had understood the risks of the study. Participants also had to indicate whether they would be willing to submit to a muscle biopsy. Exclusion criteria at this point were illnesses of heart, lung or nervous system, angina pectoris, irregularities in the stress electrocardiogram, advanced arthrosis, and hip or knee prostheses. People taking Marcumar or Sintrom (blood thinning medications) were included in the study but could not give biopsies. Participants were promised 200 francs for expenses (400 francs if they participated in the biopsies). People who did not meet the inclusion criteria could put themselves down on a waiting list. In the end, as despite great recruitment effort it became clear that the desired N of 50 could not be met under these criteria, it was decided to include people with hip or knee prostheses. To minimize the risk to their health, these participants were assigned to the cognitive training group. Group allocation was therefore no longer completely random.

Reasons for not signing up were mainly not meeting the inclusion criteria (too young, prohibitive health problems) or a stated lack of time (participants had to commit to two trainings a week for a period of three months). Several people did not sign up because allocation to treatment group was going to be random (where possible) and they were only interested in one particular type of training. The participants who had signed up for the study were then invited to an in depth health check. At the same time, they were familiarized with the physiological tests that they would later have to take at pretest (they all did a test run). 54 participants took part in this process, out of which eight were then excluded based on health check results. This left 46 participants, who were then assigned to one of three groups. As already mentioned, allocation was random where there were no health reasons prohibiting training in a specific group. Two people were allocated to the cognitive training group even though it was clear from the start that their data would have to be excluded from the final analyses. One of them had severe eye problems due to macular degeneration and the other had been examined twice before because of suspected dementia. However, as there were two free spots in this group and the two persons were very enthusiastic about the training, we decided to let these two women participate in the training and exclude their data from all analyses. Therefore, the trainings started with 16 persons in the cognitive group, and 15 persons each in the eccentric and conventional strength training group. During the three-month training period, several drop-outs occurred. In the cognitive training group, one person suffered a ruptured appendix with complications and was therefore unable to complete the training. In the strength training group, one participant did not appear regularly to the training sessions as he had just started a new relationship and preferred to invest his time there. In the eccentric training group one participant did not complete the training due to health problems. Of the people who completed the training, some data sets had to be excluded. As already mentioned, two data sets from the cognitive training group could not be used as one person had severly reduced vision and the second person was suspected to suffer from early stage dementia. Two participants in the eccentric training group suffered health problems during the training and were thus excluded (herpes zoster in one case, inflammation of the hip bursa in the second case). One additional participant in the eccentric training group had to be excluded as she did not learn to control her performance via computer screen. Hence resulted a N of 13 for the cognitive group, a N of 14 of strength training group, and a N of 11 for the eccentric training group. Thus, a total N of 38 people were included in the statistical analyses. See Figure 4 for a summary of the drop-out time line.

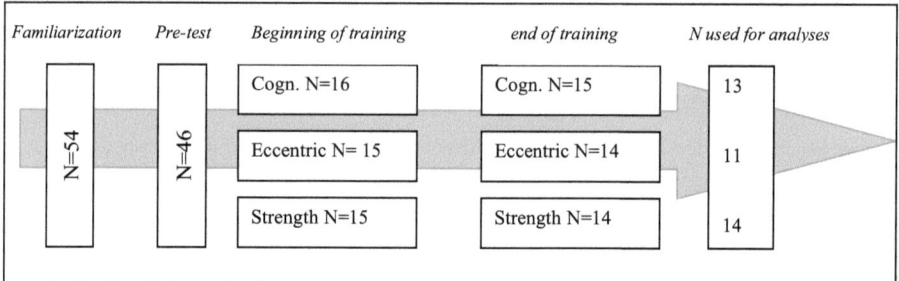

*Figure 4: Drop out time-line*

*Final Sample description*

Of the 38 people included in the final analyses, 15 were male and 23 female. Due to the lower life expectancy of males, it was despite enourmous recruitment effort impossible to find more men to participate in the study. The distribution of males and females did not differ significantly between groups (likelihood ratio $\chi^2$ (2)=1.13, $p$= .57). The mean age of the sample was 81.32 years (SD=3.37). There was no difference of mean age in the three training groups ($F(2,35)$= .38, $p$=.69) (Table 6).

*Table 6: Descriptives of sample, according to training group*

|  | Cognitive training | Eccentric training | Strength training | Total sample |
| --- | --- | --- | --- | --- |
| N | 13 | 11 | 14 | 38 |
| Age (M, *SD*) | 81.85 (*3.31*) | 81.45 (*4.01*) | 80.71 (*3.02*) | 81.32 (*3.37*) |
| Sex | 6 males, 7 females | 5 males, 6 females | 4 males, 10 females | 15 males, 23 females |

## 4.3 Description of the interventions

**Cognitive training**

As has already been mentioned in the theory part, many different training programs for the elderly exist. Most of them have focussed on improving memory by teaching strategies or mnemonics. However, the effects of these programs ususally only apply to tests that are very similar to the trained tasks. In other words, there is no generalization or transfer effects to other tasks. A second problem is that the elderly often did not use the newly learned strategies outside of the training sessions. Thirdly, most training effects tended to be short-lived. In looking for a suitable cognitive intervention program for the ExTrA study, it thus became clear that instead of using an already existing program, a new one would be created. Under the supervision of Professor Walter Perrig and in collaboration with Martin Buschkühl, a new training was designed.

It was the aim to develop a cognitive training that would yield generalized effects and would not depend on strategies, as they are rarely used outside of the laboratory. A multi-componental training was developed, with the central component being working memory training. It was hypothesized that an improvement in working memory would show widespread effects, including improvements in long-term memory and executive functions, without having to rely on strategy use.

However, as already mentioned earlier, there is some literature that suggests that cognitive performance may also be affected by negative stereotypes about aging. It was therefore decided to complement the working memory training with an activation of positive stereotypes about aging. A third component of the training was semantic activation. In this component, participants were simply shown words belonging to different categories (e.g. rivers, famous people, countries etc.). Semantic knowledge is assumed to be organized in networks. The links or connections between the different nodes of the network specify the relation between the concepts that are represented by the nodes. If one node is activated, then this activation will also spread to connected surrounding nodes. Thus, by the activation of a few nodes it is possible to activate a great amount of concepts. We assumed that the activation of nodes/concepts that had probably not been activated in a while and the resulting spread of activation to other nodes/concepts would raise the excitability of these nodes (Tranel & Damasio, 2002), and thus ease the retrieval of a great number of concepts. In view of the retrieval problems (e.g. word finding problems) reported by many elderly people, this appeared to a sensible choice for a training component.

However, it appeared crucial to us that the training would also be fun and interesting for the participants, and not just hard work. We hoped that an attractive training would ensure regular attendance and keep drop out rates low. Therefore we included two more components, which were designed not to affect memory or executive performance, but which would make the training more appealing. One of these components consisted of short presentations about different topics associated with aging and cognition (dubbed „theory"). The second component consisted of short paper-and-pencil exercises (dubbed „fun"). These fun exercises each took only 2-3 minutes and were designed not to be strenuous.

***Procedure***: Participants trained twice a week in groups of eight people. Group allocation depended on participants' schedules. One group of eight people trained Mondays and Thursdays at 2 pm, the other group trained Tuesdays and Fridays at 10 am. Both groups followed the same program. Sessions were about 50-60 minutes each and always had the same basic structure:
Participants usually arrived early and discussed their homework of the previous session. After everybody had arrived, each session started with a short description of what would happen in this day's session. Participants then worked on computers for about 20 minutes (the computer block contained the working memory training, stereotype activation as well as semantic activation, and will be described in more detail in the next paragraph). After that, they seated themselves around a table for a theory block of about 10-15 minutes. Usually, a lively discussion ensued at the end of this block, which was often continued for another half hour over tea and coffee. During this time, participants also exchanged stories, chatted or shared problems (e.g. with hearing aids, moving). Participants received a short written summary of the theory (less than a page) at the end of each session, together with voluntary homework. At each training session, two instructors were present (with very few exceptions due to illness, they were always the same two persons), with one instructor having the lead and the second person supporting. The training room contained eight computers in the back (set up in two rows facing the side walls) and a big table with chairs in the front.

***Description of the computer block***: Each computer block included several tasks. All tasks were programmed on eprime (Schneider, Eschman, & Zuccolotto, 2002) and presented on Windows computers with 15" screens. The reaction time task was programmed by myself; the other tasks were programmed by M. Buschkühl. Each computer block contained a semantic activation, a stereotype activation, a working memory task, followed by another stereotype activation and, finally, another session of semantic activation. The following tasks were used over the 23 sessions (to see which tasks were used in which sessions, please see Appendix 1):

- *Flower-Task*

As the majority of the partipants was not familiar with computers, the first session was dedicated to getting to know and getting comfortable with the computer. This included practising using the mouse. The flower task was designed especially for this purpose. In this task, pictures of flowers were arranged in a circle on the screen. One picture would then be replaced by a red field, and the participant had to move the arrow with the mouse to that spot as fast as possible and click on it. The computer then displayed a feedback about the reaction time, and another flower would be replaced by red, etc.

- *Semantic activation*

With exception of the first session, each computer block started and ended with semantic activation. In this task, participants were shown 76 words. 48 of these words were adjectives, the other 28 words stemmed from four different categories (i.e. seven words per category). The words were shown for a duration of at least 2000 milliseconds. If a word was longer than eight letters, the duration was extended by 150 miliseconds per additional letter. Participants were instructed to sit comfortably and just attentively read the words, and not try to memorize them.

- *Reaction time task*

In the reaction time task, participants were presented a screen with a fixation cross, followed by a word which was shown for 115ms and then immediately covered by a mask of consonants. None of the participants ever mentioned seeing anything before the mask. The mask remained onscreen until the participant's reaction. The word respectively the mask would appear either above or underneath a fixation cross which would disappear at the word's presentation. The participants' task was to press the „Y" key if the word/mask was placed above the fixation cross, and to press the „M" key if the word/mask appeared underneath. Each session contained two reaction time tasks. In this task, participants were presented with positive stereotypes about aging before the appearance of the mask. These stereotypes/words had been selected as follows (procedure analogous to Levy, 1996): 10 people of different ages (from 25 to 55) were asked to write down positive sentences about aging or old people. The keywords of these sentences (e.g. wise) were then rated by five other people (aged 26-58) in regard to how representative they are for old age and also in regard to positive valence. There resulted a list of twelve words which were consistently rated as representative for old age and positive. These words were then presented in five runs, with the presentation order following Levy (1996). Each run began with either the word „*alt*" or „*Senior*". Then followed the twelve stereotypes (*weise, ruhig, Freizeit, erfahren, Wissen, zufrieden, Zuneigung, geduldig, freundlich, ausgeglichen, genügsam, liebenswürdig*) in different order, interspersed with four neutral words (*zusammen, Satz, zwischen* and *andere*r). Two of the stereotypes, weise (wise) and erfahren (experienced) were presented twice, as was the first word (alt or Senior; however, this word could not appear at second, second-to-last or last position).

- *Lexical decision task*

In the lexical decision tasks, participants were presented with sequences of letters and had to decide whether the sequence actually made up a word or was a non-word. Participants had to press the Y key if it was a word and the M key if the letter sequence was a non-word. The words used in this task were the same ones as used in the reaction time task. The letter sequences remained onscreen until the participant's answer.

- *Senso*

Four colorful squares (red, green, yellow and blue) were displayed on the screen. These squares would then blink in a certain order. Participants had to memorize that order and then replicate it by clicking (with the mouse) on the relevant squares in the right order. The number of squares to be memorized increased if participants successfully replicated a sequence. However, if participants made a mistake, the number of squares to be remembered decreased by one. It was thus an adaptive task.

- *Cats&Dogs task (C&D)*

The cats and dogs task consisted of two parts. In the first part, participants were shown a picture of either a dog or a cat and had to decide whether this picture was presented upside down or the right way around. Pressing the right mouse key indicated that the picture was presented correctly, whereas pressing the left mouse key indicated that the picture was upside down. Responses had to be correct and occurr within 3000 milliseconds, otherwise a message appeared on screen to remind the participants to answer correctly and as quickly as possible. The task continued only after participants had corrected previously wrong answers. In the second part, participants had to remember the sequence of cats and dogs, e.g. cat – dog – cat – cat. Whether the pictures had been upside down or not did not matter anymore at this stage. The participants could enter the sequence by using the mouse to click on the pictures of a cat and a dog. This task was also adaptive. First, participants were only presented with two pictures. Not only did the order have to be correctly replicated to proceed to the next level but also the decision upside down or not had to be correct and occur within a certain time. The cats and dogs task proved to be quite challenging, as two things had to be done at the same time: Decide upon the position of the picture as well as remember the order of cats and dogs.

- *Animal span*

The animal span task was a further development of the cats & dogs task. Instead of just one cat and one dog, there were eight animals all in all, a cat, a dog (different from the ones used in the cats & dogs task), an iguana, a toad, a bunny, a butterfly, a rat and a bee. All pictures were in color. Apart from the bigger selection of animals, the task was identical to the cats & dogs task.

It is important to note that not all tasks were used in each session. The flower task, for example, was only used in the first few sessions to familiarize participants with the computer. The senso task was only used in the first third of the sessions, and was then relaced with first the cats & dogs task and later with the animal span task. Semantic activation and either the reaction time task or the lexical decision task were used in every session apart from the very first one. For a detailed description on which task was used in which session, please consult appendix 1.

***Description of the theory block***: In this block, participants were given information about various topics related to cognition, like memory, attention, the visual system etc. A detailed list of the topics covered can be found in appendix II. It is important to note that no mnemonics were taught, apart from a technique to memorize people's names in the first lesson. At the end of each session, participants were given a written summary of the theory covered in that particular session.

***Description of the voluntary homework***: At the beginning of the study it was planned that ten minutes of each session would be devoted to fun exercises. These exercises were specifically chosen to not influence memory performance. The purpose was to provide a short time which would not be performance-oriented but mainly fun. However, it turned out that usually too much time was taken up by the theory part and the ensuing disussion to leave room for the „fun part". As the participants highly valued the theory and the discussion, we decided to turn the „fun part" into voluntary homework. Thus, at the end of each session the participants received some fun exercises. It was stressed that these exercises were voluntary. However, all the participants almost always completed the exercises. Solutions to the exercises were distributed at the beginning of the next lesson. Great care was taken that no participant should feel exposed had s/he made a mistake; this included that the leaders did not ask who had made mistakes and did not check the participants' homework unless requested. For examples of the exercises please refer to appendix III.

## Eccentric training

The eccentric training was designed and led by Professor Hoppeler from the Institut of Anatomy, University of Bern, and his team. Eccentric muscle training denotes training while the muscle is lengthening (as opposed to concentric muscle training, where the muscle contracts). An everyday example of eccentric muscle activity is walking down the stairs (while walking up the stairs involves concentric muscle activity). The muscle lengthening while the muscle works is called eccentric contraction. Eccentric contractions are associated with lower metabolic and cardiovascular cost than concentric contractions, but nevertheless cause strength gains and increase in muscle mass (Hortobagyi, Money, Zheng, Dudek, Fraser, & Dohm 2002). Eccentric exercise may thus be especially well suited for elderly persons, which is one reason why it was chosen in the ExTrA study.

Each training session started with a questionnaire to assess delayed onset of muscle soreness (DOMS-score) of the last training session. After that, a warm-up followed to minimize the risk of injuries. The actual training took place on a computer-controlled eccentric cycle ergometer. At first view, this ergometer resembles a bike with the pedals in front of the participant and an elevated computer screen. The pedals move backwards, driven by a motor. The task for the participant is to resist this motor driven movement with a specific amount of force („braking"). The computer screen displays a curve of the braking effort, which is to be used by the participant as feedback. The amplitude of this curve is supposed to stay within certain limits, clearly marked with two horizontal lines. It demanded divided attention to regulate one's force application while watching the screen. The physical activity targeted the knee extensor muscles (M. vastus lateralis).

Participants started out with 5 minutes eccentric training time per session, which was then increased stepwise (5 minutes increase per session) up to 20 minutes total training time. Not only training duration, but also training intensity was successively ramped (up to 70% of the maximal individual heart rate). The heart rate was monitored continuously, and each participant was coached one-on-one. At the end of each session, participants completed a rating of perceived exertion (BORG-score).

## Conventional strength training

As opposed to the eccentric training group, the second training group used a more conventional training, such as can be found in fitness centers. This training consisted mainly of concentric muscle activity, and involved the following four exercises: Leg press, knee extension, one leg hip extension left, and one leg hip extension right. All these exercises were performed on weight machines in a fitness center. This training was also led by the team of Professor Hoppeler.
Just like in the eccentric training group, each training session started with a questionnaire to assess delayed onset of muscle soreness (DOMS-score) of the last training session. After that followed a warm up which involved especially ankle, knee and hip joints. During the first four training sessions, participants then started with one warm up set followed by one full power set with 12-15 repetitions for each exercise. From the fifth session on, the warm-up set was followed by two full power sets. Whenever a participant managed to do more than 12 repetitions, the load (i.e. weight resistance) was increased. At the end of the training everybody participated in a 5 minute cool-down, and then completed a rating of perceived exertion (BORG-score). The training was conducted in groups of four people, with an instructor present at all times. Just like in the eccentric training, the strength training was also designed to target the extensor muscles of the knee.

All three trainings were designed to take the same amount of time per week (i.e. 45 minutes). Group sizes differed between the different trainings because of situational constraints (only one eccentric cycle ergometer, not enough room for more than 8 computers in the cognitive training group, not enough training stations for more than four people in the strength training group). Pre-, post- and follow-up testing were identical for all participants, no matter which group they belonged to. These test procedures will now be examined in more detail.

## 4.4 Assessment

The testing for each participant took place over two consecutive days. On the first day, participants started with a one-hour psychology testing block. After completing that block, they had a fifteen minute break before moving on to another hour of physiological testing. On the second day, participants returned for another hour's psychological testing session. Both pre- and posttest took place in the same venue, and all the tests (psychological and physiological) were done in a one-to-one setting. The order of tests was identical for each participant. Great care was taken to make the participants feel comfortable. There was always one person designated to welcome people, offer them something to drink and to eat and chat with them until the testing (or the next phase of testing in the fifteen-minute break) started. A list of all test used and their order of presentation is displayed in Table 7. In the following section, only those measures that were pertinent to this thesis will be described in more detail, starting with the cognitive measures.

*Table 7: List of test instruments used in the psychological assessement*

| Test | Author(s) |
|---|---|
| **Testing on first day** | |
| NAA (adapted, combined with IDA) | Fleischmann & Oswald (1997-1999) |
| Health related control beliefs | Perrig-Chiello, Perrig & Staehelin (1999) |
| WHOQOL-Bref | Angermeyer, Kilian & Matschinger (2000) |
| Prospective memory | proprietary development (with W.J. Perrig and M. Buschkühl) |
| Digit Symbol Test (taken from NAI) | Fleischmann & Oswald (1997-1999) |
| Digit Span (taken from HAWIE-R) | Tewes (2001) |
| VS 2 | proprietary development (programmed by M. Buschkühl), based on article by Klingberg, Forssberg & Westerberg, 2002 |
| Stroop (taken from NAI) | Fleischmann & Oswald (1997-1999) |
| Morningness /Eveningness Questionnaire | |
| **Testing on second day** | |
| Prospective memory (continuation) | proprietary development |
| MWT | Lehrl (1989); Lehrl, Merz, Burkhard & Fischer (1991) |
| Wechsler Memory Story (taken from WMS-R) | Härting et al. (2000) |
| C-GFT<br>    Test of vision<br>    Estimation of one's own memory<br>    finding the differences<br>    Clarification<br>    Attention (Sun-Task)<br>    Dual Task (Sun task and Clarification)<br>    Free Recall (objects in picture)<br>    Free Recall (differences between pict.)<br>    Attribution of performance<br>    Recognition | Perrig et al. (1994) |
| Wechsler Memory Story (Free Recall) | Härting et al. (2000) |
| *only at posttest: Questionnaire of subjectively experienced change* | proprietary development |

### 4.4.1 Cognitive measures

An overview of all the measures used, the cognitive function they purport to measure and the measures' origins are displayed in Table 8. The measures will be grouped according to cognitive function.

**Speed:**
- The ZS-G from the *Nürnberger Altersinventar NAI* (Fleischmann & Oswald, 1997-1999) is a test analogous to the Digit-Symbol Test of the Wechsler Adult Intelligence Scale (WAIS), only in bigger print and with different symbols. On top of the page there are the numbers 1-9, each with a different symbol beneath it. In the lower part of the page follow rows with numbers. The participants have to put as many of the appropriate symbols underneath each number as they can manage within 90 seconds. The retest reliabilty of this test is $r_{tt}$= .89 - .97 (after a four to twelve week re-test-interval). There are norm values from a sample of 1424 healthy participants between 55 and 95 years.
- *Reaction time* task, taken from the "Computergestützter Gedächtnisfunktionstest" (Computer-supported test of memory function, Perrig et al., 1994). In this test, Participants have to react to suns appearing either on right or the left hand side of the computer screen by pressing either the left or the right mouse button. The test is reported to be reliable (Kling, 1996).

**Executive functions:**
- *Farb-Wort-Test (Color-Word Interference Test)*, taken from the NAI: This test is analogous to the Stroop test (Baeumler, 1985), with the difference that everything is printed in a much bigger font appropriate for older people. In a first run, participants have to read out loud a table of words denoting colors (blue, green, red, yellow) as fast as possible. These words are printed in black. The second task is to name the color of little swathes of color printed on a sheet as quickly as possible (again, the colors are blue, green, red, and yellow). The third task combines tasks one and two. This time, the words blue, green, yellow and red are printed in those colors; however, the written word and the color do not correspond (e.g. blue will be written in red ink, etc.). The task is to name as quickly as possible the colors the words are printed with, and to inhibit the automatic reading reaction. The retest-reliability for the tasks II and III, $r_{tt}$, lies between .74 and .89 (after an interval of 5-8 weeks). The interference value calculated by subtracting the time used for task two from the time used for task three is reported to have a

retest reliability of between .70 and .83 (Fleischmann & Oswald, 1997-1999). This interference value was chosen as a measure of inhibition.

- Dual task (taken from C-GFT): In this task, the reaction time task described above is combined with having to identify blurry pictures that become progressively clearer in the middle of the computer screen. The number of suns that were correctly reacted to despite this distraction constitute the measure *"Dual task hits"*. The mean reaction time to the suns constitute the measure *"Dual task reaction time"*. Both of these tasks measure task coordination, which is an executive function. The test is considered reliable (see Kling 1996).

**Memory:**

- *Zahlennachsprechen ZN-G (Digit Span Test)*, taken from NAI: This test is analogous to the digit span subtest of the WAIS. Participants are orally presented with an increasingly long sequence of digits, which they have to repeat back to the interviewer, in a first task in the same order, then, in a second task, backwards. The ZN-G is considered a „task of medium reliability", as retest-reliability is reported to be around $r_{tt}$ = .60 (Fleischmann & Oswald, 1997-1999). The ZN-G forward score was taken to represent short-term memory span, while the ZN-G backwards score was taken as an indicator of working memory.

- *WMS*: One task was taken from the german version of the Wechsler Memory scale (Härting et al., 2000) and slightly modified. Instead of orally presenting two stories, we used only one; furthermore, there was no immediate recall, only a delayed one. Retest-reliability for the original version is reported to be .79 (Härting et al., 2000). The WMS score was used as a measure of long-term episodic memory.

- *Free Recall and Recognition (C-GFT):* Participants have to identify the differences between to pictures that appear identical at first sight. At the same time, however, they are instructed to memorize the objects depicted in the drawing. Several tasks later, participants are asked to recall which objects they had seen in that drawing. Correctly recalled items from this task constitute the *"free recall"* measure. Finally, participants are presented with a sheet with a number of items and have to identify those items that were part of the original drawing. Correctly identified items make up the *"recognition"* measure (note: it could be argued that a recognition discrimination measure, d', would be better suited to measure the actual recognition performance. All analyses were therefore also computed with d'; however, none of these analyses reached significance). Both the free recall and the recognition tasks were used as indicators of visual long-term memory. Retest-reliability is reported to be .64 for Free Recall and .49 for Recognition (Meier & Perrig, 2000).

*Table 8: Overview of tests used to assess cognitive functioning*

| Cognitive function | | Assessed by | Test Origin | Abbreviation |
|---|---|---|---|---|
| Speed | | Digit-Symbol-Test | NAI | DST |
| | | Reaction time task | C-GFT | RT |
| Executive functions | inhibition | Stroop test | NAI | Strp |
| | task coordination | Dual task hits | C-GFT | DT$_{hits}$ |
| | | Dual task reaction time | C-GFT | DT$_{rt}$ |
| Memory | memory span | Digit Span forward | NAI | DS $_{forward}$ |
| | working memory | Digit Span backward | NAI | DS $_{backward}$ |
| | episodic memory (verbal) | Wechsler Story | WMS | WMS |
| | episodic memory (visual) | Free Recall, Recognition | C-GFT | FreeRec, Recog |

### 4.4.2 Well-being measures

The well-being measure used in the ExTrA study was the german short version of the World Health Organization Quality of life Questionnaire (WHOQOL-Bref, Angermeyer et al., 2000). Even though the instrument is, according to the name, supposed to assess quality of life, the authors state that they aim to assess „the individual perception of one's own living situation in the context of the respective culture and values and in relation to one's own goals, expectations, standards and interests " (translated from Angermeyer et al., 2000, p. 10). Even though several questions refer to "objective" topics such as concentration or housing, the questionnaire always assesses the participant's subjective evaluation respectively satisfaction with it (eleven of twenty-six items start with "how satisfied are you with ..."). Therefore, in terms of the conceptualization of quality of life and well-being given earlier, the WHOQOL-Bref measures well-being (which also contains satisfaction measures) rather than quality of life. Therefore, it was decided that it is acceptable to use this test as a measure of well-being.

The WHOQOL-Bref was given at both pre- and posttest. It encompasses five domains of well-being: Physical, psychological, social relationships, environment, and global. The items of each domain are displayed in

Table 9. The sum of all subscales was taken as an indicator of overall well-being. Difference values (posttest minus pretest scores) were interpreted as indicators of improvement.

The questionnaire was conducted as an interview rather than given to the participants to fill out by themselves. The possible answer options for each item were laid out successively in front of the participants as a memory help. The WHOQOL-Bref was given quite early in each examination, after an assessment of daily activities and health-related control beliefs, which took approximately ten minutes altogether.

*Table 9: Domains and items of the WHOQOL-BREF*

| | WHOQOL-BREF | | | | |
|---|---|---|---|---|---|
| **domain** | physical | psychological | social | environment | global |
| **items** | pain | positive feelings | personal relationships | physical safety | quality of life in general |
| | energy | learning / memory / concentration | sexual activity | home environment | satisfaction with health |
| | sleep | self-esteem | social support | financial resources | |
| | mobility | body image | | health care accessibility | |
| | activities of daily living | negative feelings | | opportunity for acquiring information | |
| | dependence on medical substances | spirituality / religion | | opportunity for leisure activities | |
| | work capacity | | | physical environment | |
| | | | | transport | |

*Reliability and validity of the WHOQOL-Bref:* The reliability coefficients for all subscales are higher than .70 (non-clinical sample of 2000 german-speaking persons), and is thus acoording to the authors „acceptable" (Angermeyer et al., 2000). Content validity is assumed to be the same as in the longer version of the questionnaire, the WHOQOL-100, which was considered satisfactory. Construct validity is described as excellent (Angermeyer et al., 2000).

## 4.5 Statistical analyses

All statistical analyses were computed with the SPSS software package for Mac OS X, Version 11. Dependent variables were tested for normality distribution with the Shapiro-Wilks rather than the Kolmogorov-Smirnov-test, as the Shapiro-Wilks is reported to be more accurate (Field, 2005, p. 545), and better suited to small samples. Homogeneity of variance was assessed prior to all analyses with the Levene-Test. If the assumption of normal distribution and homogeneity of variance was violated, non-parametric analyses were used instead of parametric ones.

Repeated measures analyses of variance were computed for all variables, followed by planned contrasts if there was a specific hypothesis (repeated measures were also computed on non-parametric data, as there is no non-parametric equivalent). To examine pre-post differences within one group, the Wilcoxon test for non-parametric data or a paired samples t-test for parametric data was used. For reporting Wilcoxon results, it was decided to present Median scores, z- and p- values as well as r as an indicator of effect size (in accordance with Field, 2005). In some cases, where the Median scores were misleading, mean scores were presented additionally. In cases where there were baseline differences between groups, ANCOVAs were computed with the posttest scores as dependent variable and the pretest scores as covariates. Power analyses were conducted with help of the G*Power program (Buchner, Faul, & Erdfelder, 1997).

## 4.6 Hypotheses

### 4.6.1 Hypotheses concerned with cognition

A study by Klingberg, Forssberg and Westerberg (2002) has shown that working memory training has a positive effect on working memory capacity as well as other cognitive measures. This study was conducted with children and young adults. However, in view of the very strong evidence that many different aspects of cognition in the elderly are trainable, it can be assumed that a working memory training would also have benefits in a sample of older participants. Furthermore, it has also been shown that cognitive restructuring can have positive effects on memory performance (e.g. Levy, 1996). Seeing as the cognitive training used in the ExTrA study contained both working memory training and cognitive restructuring, an improvement of memory can be expected. The working memory training was a dual task, therefore, an improvement in executive functions is also expected. In addition to working memory training and cognitive restructuring, the training contained also a reaction time training. Even though the task used at pre- and posttest was not identical to the task used in training, there is enough similarity between the two tasks to expect a positive training effect.

Meta-analyses have shown that physical training has a positive effect on cognition in the elderly (e.g. Colcombe & Kramer, 2003), especially on executive functions. As the eccentric training used in the ExTrA study contained certain dual task aspects (watching a monitor while nonstop adjusting one's use of strength on the ergometer), it is expected that the improvement in executive functions will be bigger in the eccentric training group than in the conventional strength training group. Several studies have also reported physical exercise effects on speed (e.g. Dustman et al., 1984; Stones & Kozma, 1996). However, Perrig-Chiello et al. (1998) did not find any improvement in speed after eight weeks of resistance training. Therefore, we expect a pre-posttest improvement in speed only in the eccentric exercise group. The same study did, however, find an improvement in memory for resistance training, which is why the conventional strength training is expected to yield certain gains in memory functioning. Based on this reasoning, the following hypotheses are formulated (the hypotheses are grouped according to type of training and not psychological function, as the comparison of different trainings and not certain cognitive functions are the main theme of this thesis):

**Hypotheses regarding eccentric training:** The eccentric training intervention leads to an improvement in speed und executive functions, but not in memory.

**Hypotheses regarding conventional strength training:** The conventional strength training intervention leads to an improvement in executive functions und memory, but not in speed.

**Hypotheses regarding cognitive training:** The cognitive training group will show a pre-posttest improvement in memory, speed, and executive functions, even though the tasks used at pre- and posttest were not practiced during the intervention (transfer effects).

**Hypotheses comparing the effects of the different types of training:**
1. The improvement in executive functions is smaller in the conventional training group than in the eccentric exercise group.
2. The cognitive training group shows the greatest improvement in executive functions of all three training groups.
3. Cognitive training is more effective in improving memory performance than either eccentric or conventional strength training.

In addition to these hypotheses, it was also of interest whether age, intelligence, gender, or baseline performance would be associated with subsequent improvement or decline. These questions will be examined after the hypotheses.

## 4.6.2 Hypotheses concerned with well-being

Several reviews and meta-analyses of the past few years come to the conlusion that there is an association between physical exercise and psychological well-being (Arent et al., 2000; McAuley & Rudolph, 1995; Netz et al., 2005; Spirduso & Cronin, 2001). Even though the results of correlational and prospective longitudinal studies have yielded stronger evidence of such an association than intervention studies, there is nevertheless sufficient evidence that a physical exercise intervention may have positive effects on well-being. In contrast, the evidence of a similar link between cognitive training and well-being is still lacking. However, there is a wealth of studies showing that cognitive training can lead to an improvement in cognitive function (e.g. Oswald et al., 1996; Scogin et al., 1985; Stigsdotter Neely & Bäckman, 1995). Seeing as Jones and colleagues (2003) found that cognitive functioning is predicitive of life satisfaction and positive affect, two aspects that are generally considered to be crucial aspects of well-being, one can assume that cognitive training is likely to have a positive influence on well-being by way of improving cognitive functioning. Additionally, the cognitive training intervention included an activation of positive attitudes about aging, which may also improve well-being. However, considering the wealth of evidence that support a positive effect of physical training in comparison to the lack of evidence regarding cognitive training, it is assumed that the effect of physical training yields a stronger effect than cognitive training.

Up to this point, no study has assessed the influence of eccentric exercise on well-being. It is therefore difficult to make a theory-guided prediction whether eccentric exercise is more or less beneficial for well-being than traditional strength training. However, based on the fact that eccentric exercise is usually experienced as less strenuous or taxing than other forms of exercise, this may lead to less experience of mastery, which has been associated with well-being. Therefore it is assumed that eccentric exercise will have a smaller effect on well-being than traditional strength training.

Last but not least, it is of interest whether changes in cognition were predictive of changes in well-being. As memory complaints are the most frequently voiced complaints of older people in regard to cognition, it is possible that an improvement in cognition would be associated with an increase in well-being. However, according to literature, it is not necessarily to be expected that change in memory is predictive of change in well-being, as several studies have found that an increase in cognitive function was not accompanied by an increase in well-being.

**Physical training hypotheses**: Physical training leads to an increase in overall well-being. Furthermore, on the domain level, physical training leads to an improvement in physical and psychological well-being. However, the improvement is greater in physical well-being.

**Cognitive training hypotheses**: Cognitive training leads to an increase in both physical and psychological well-being: The increase in psychological well-being is expected to be greater than the one in physical well-being.

**Hypotheses concerned with training comparisons:**
1. Both physical training as well as cognitive training leads to an improvement in total amount of well-being; however, the improvement is greater in the physical training groups.
2. Conventional strength training has a greater positive effect on physical and psychological well-being than eccentric strength training.

**Hypothesis concerned with the interrelation of cognition and well-being**: An improvement in memory variables is predictive of an improvement in overall well-being.

# 5 Results

The results section will be divided into two parts. The first part will display the results concerned with cognition, while the second part will focus on the results concerned with well-being. Each part will begin with a section on means and standard deviations of the measures used, followed by distribution testing, pre-posttest correlations, pre-posttest differences, and group differences at prestest (baseline differences). After that follow the results of the hypothesis testing.

## 5.1 Cognition

### 5.1.1 Descriptives, distribution testing, correlations

*Descriptives*: The means and standard deviations of all cognitive measures used in the hypotheses, grouped according to training intervention, can be found in Table 10.

*Distribution testing:* Skewness and kurtosis of all cognitive pretest and posttest scores were within acceptable range (i.e. below 2.58, as recommended by Field, 2005, for small samples). At pretest, the Digit Span scores, Stroop inhibition scores, Reaction time, Free recall as well as recognition scores deviated significantly from normal distribution (Shapiro-Wilks, all $ps < .05$). The digit-symbol scores, Wechsler Memory scores, as well as the Dual task scores, were normally distributed (Shapiro-Wilks, all $ps > .05$).

For all pretest scores, distribution testing was also conducted according to training group. These computations yielded that Stroop scores, all Digit Span subtest scores, as well as Free recall scores deviated in one or several groups from normal distribution (Shapiro-Wilks, $ps < .05$). The other scores were normally distributed.

At posttest, the Digit span scores, reaction time, dual task hits and free recall scores deviated significantly from normal distribution (Shapiro-Wilks, all $ps \leq .05$). All other scores were normally distributed.

Distribution testing was also conducted for pre-posttest difference scores. The difference values of digit span forwards, digit span total score, stroop inhibition, reaction time as well as dual task reaction time differed significantly from normal distribution (Shapiro-Wilks, all $ps < .05$), all other scores were normally distributed.

*Pre-posttest correlations:* Spearman's rho was used to compute correlations between pre- and posttest scores for all Digit span subtests, Stroop inhibition scores, rection time, dual task hits, Free recall, and recognition, as these measures were not normally distributed at pre- and/or posttest. Pre-Posttest correlations for Digit symbol Test, Wechsler Memory, and Dual Task reaction time were computed with Pearson correlations. All correlations are listed in Table 11. All pretest scores correlated significantly with the posttest scores, with the exception of the C-GFT Recognition measure. This measure failed to show a significant pre-posttest correlation. Therefore, in most cases, a certain test-retest reliablity was confirmed by our data.

*Table 10: Descriptives of cognitive variables at pre- and posttest*

|  | Cognitive Training | | Conven. Strength Training | | Eccentric Strength Training | | baseline differences |
|---|---|---|---|---|---|---|---|
|  | M | SD | M | SD | M | SD |  |
| *n* | 13 | | 14 | | 11 | | |
| **Digit Symbol Test** | | | | | | | |
| *Pretest* | 36.69 | 8.19 | 37.00 | 7.08 | 36.73 | 8.32 | .994 |
| *Posttest* | 37.62 | 7.02 | 39.86 | 7.65 | 37.55 | 5.94 | |
| **Digit Span forw** | | | | | | | |
| *Pretest* | 5.38 | 0.77 | 5.79 | 1.05 | 6.36 | 0.67 | .026* |
| *Posttest* | 5.31 | 0.63 | 6.00 | 0.68 | 6.09 | 0.70 | |
| **Digit Span back** | | | | | | | |
| *Pretest* | 4.23 | 1.09 | 4.57 | 1.40 | 4.82 | 0.75 | .384 |
| *Posttest* | 4.15 | 1.14 | 4.50 | 0.94 | 4.64 | 1.03 | |
| **Digit Span total** | | | | | | | |
| *Pretest* | 9.62 | 1.33 | 10.36 | 2.06 | 11.18 | 1.08 | .031* |
| *Posttest* | 9.46 | 1.26 | 10.50 | 1.29 | 10.73 | 1.01 | |
| **Stroop inh.** | | | | | | | |
| *Pretest* | 29.62 | 12.84 | 22.43 | 7.50 | 20.45 | 6.47 | .076 |
| *Posttest* | 22.84 | 8.76 | 18.99 | 7.31 | 22.20 | 6.45 | |
| **Wechsler Memory Story** | | | | | | | |
| *Pretest* | 10.23 | 3.42 | 9.07 | 3.81 | 10.55 | 4.13 | .584 |
| *Posttest* | 8.46 | 4.31 | 8.07 | 3.43 | 10.27 | 2.24 | |
| **Reaction Time** | | | | | | | |
| *Pretest* | 0.41 | 0.02 | 0.41 | 0.06 | 0.44 | 0.08 | .264 |
| *Posttest* | 0.42 | 0.05 | 0.43 | 0.09 | 0.42 | 0.06 | |
| **Dual task hits** | | | | | | | |
| *Pretest* | 75.90 | 13.71 | 77.49 | 10.31 | 87.11 | 7.66 | .039* |
| *Posttest* | 77.54 | 19.72 | 81.30 | 13.97 | 90.11 | 8.31 | |
| **Dual task RT** | | | | | | | |
| *Pretest* | 0.46 | 0.09 | 0.48 | 0.09 | 0.48 | 0.08 | .829 |
| *Posttest* | 0.52 | 0.07 | 0.46 | 0.11 | 0.46 | 0.06 | |
| **Free Recall** | | | | | | | |
| *Pretest* | 6.15 | 2.73 | 5.64 | 4.81 | 5.27 | 2.72 | .438 |
| *Posttest* | 7.69 | 3.75 | 6.64 | 4.36 | 5.64 | 2.80 | |
| **Recognition** | | | | | | | |
| *Pretest* | 11.54 | 2.63 | 12.07 | 2.95 | 9.73 | 3.23 | .138 |
| *Posttest* | 11.46 | 3.41 | 9.86 | 3.46 | 9.36 | 2.62 | |

\* $p < .05$

*Correlations between the measures at pretest*

The pretest correlations between the different cognitive measures are listed in Table 13. Non-parametric correlations were computed with Spearman's rho, the parametric ones with the Pearson correlation coefficient. The correlation matrix largely confirms the grouping of variables done in the hypotheses part (it was not possible to compute a factor analysis due to the small sample size). For example, the two measures postulated to assess speed, i.e. reaction time and digit symbol test, show a significant correlation, as do the two measures postulated to measure executive function, Stroop and Dual task hits. The one area where measures do not correlate significantly is memory. However, this can be explained with the fact that the different tests assess very different types of memory. Digit span, as the name already implies, is a measure of memory span (i.e. short term memory), the Wechsler Memory story assesses verbal episodic memory (more long-term), while the Free Recall and Recognition measures taken from the C-GFT estimate visual memory.

*- Correlations between cognitive and well-being measures at pretest*

There are almost no significant correlations between cognitive and well-being measures at pretest. Only three correlations reach significance. Digit Span forwards correlates significantly with the WHOQOL-psychological subscale ($\rho = -.430$, $p = .007$), as does Dual Task reaction time ($r = -.401$, $p = .013$), and Wechsler memory correlates significantly with the WHOQOL global subscale ($\rho = .417$, $p = .009$). There were no other significant correlations (all $ps > .05$).

*Table 11: Correlations between non-parametric pretest and posttest scores of the different cognitive measures*

| Pretest | | Posttest | | | | | | | |
|---|---|---|---|---|---|---|---|---|---|
| | | Digit Span forward | Digit Span backward | Digit Span total | Stroop inhibition | cgft - Reaction | cgft - Recognition | cgft - Free Recall | Dual task hits |
| Digit Span forward | Rho<br>Sig. | .481**<br>.002 | | | | | | | |
| Digit Span backward | Rho<br>Sig. | | .342*<br>.035 | | | | | | |
| Digit Span total | Rho<br>Sig. | | | .535**<br>.001 | | | | | |
| Stroop inhibition | Rho<br>Sig. | | | | .684**<br>.000 | | | | |
| cgft - Reaction | Rho<br>Sig. | | | | | .402*<br>.012 | | | |
| cgft – Recogn. | Rho<br>Sig. | | | | | | .194<br>.242 | | |
| cgft - Free Recall | Rho<br>Sig. | | | | | | | .529**<br>.001 | |
| Dual Task hits | Rho<br>Sig. | | | | | | | | .661**<br>.000 |

** Correlation is significant at the .01 level (2-tailed).
* Correlation is significant at the .05 level (2-tailed).

*Table 12: Correlations between parametric pretest and posttest scores of the different cognitive measures*

| Pretest | | Posttest | | |
|---|---|---|---|---|
| | | Digit Symbol Test | Wechsler Memory | Dual Task RT |
| Digit Symbol Test | Pearson corr<br>Sig. (2-tailed) | .764**<br>.000 | | |
| Wechsler Memory | Pearson corr<br>Sig. (2-tailed) | | .432**<br>.007 | |
| Dual Task RT | Pearson corr<br>Sig. (2-tailed) | | | .360*<br>.026 |

** Correlation is significant at the .01 level (2-tailed).
* Correlation is significant at the .05 level (2-tailed).

Table 13: Correlations between cognitive measures at pretest

Pretest

| Pretest | | Digit Span forward | Digit Span backward | Digit Span total | Stroop inhibition | cgft - Reaction | cgft - Recognition | cgft - Free Recall | Dual Task hits | Digit Symbol Test | Wechsler Memory | Dual task RT |
|---|---|---|---|---|---|---|---|---|---|---|---|---|
| Digit Span forward | Rho | - | .251 | .758** | -.149 | .193 | .179 | -.022 | .175 | .148 | -.098 | -.139 |
| | Sig. (2-tailed) | - | .129 | .000 | .373 | .246 | .281 | .896 | .294 | .377 | .558 | .407 |
| Digit Span backward | Rho | | - | .794** | -.182 | -.045 | .026 | -.135 | .178 | .662** | .065 | -.056 |
| | Sig. (2-tailed) | | - | .000 | .275 | .790 | .876 | .417 | .284 | .000 | .696 | .738 |
| Digit Span total | Rho | | | - | -.224 | .129 | .116 | -.072 | .240 | .517** | -.062 | -.066 |
| | Sig. (2-tailed) | | | - | .177 | .439 | .489 | .669 | .147 | .001 | .709 | .693 |
| Stroop inhibition | Rho | | | | - | .134 | -.109 | .169 | -.334* | -.419** | -.213 | .084 |
| | Sig. (2-tailed) | | | | - | .421 | .513 | .311 | .040 | .009 | .200 | .614 |
| cgft - Reaction | Rho | | | | | - | .076 | .163 | -.249 | -.388* | .029 | .320* |
| | Sig. (2-tailed) | | | | | - | .649 | .329 | .132 | .016 | .861 | .050 |
| cgft – Recogn. | Rho | | | | | | - | .266 | -.128 | .183 | -.101 | -.161 |
| | Sig. (2-tailed) | | | | | | - | .106 | .442 | .270 | .546 | .335 |
| cgft - Free Recall | Rho | | | | | | | - | .117 | -.067 | .051 | -.099 |
| | Sig. (2-tailed) | | | | | | | - | .483 | .690 | .760 | .556 |
| Dual Task hits | Rho | | | | | | | | - | .422** | .141 | -.215 |
| | Sig. (2-tailed) | | | | | | | | - | .008 | .397 | .195 |
| Digit Symbol Test | Rho | | | | | | | | | - | .182 | -.286 |
| | Sig. (2-tailed) | | | | | | | | | - | .275 | .082 |
| Wechsler Memory | Rho | | | | | | | | | | - | -.286 |
| | Sig. (2-tailed) | | | | | | | | | | - | .082 |
| Dual task RT | Rho | | | | | | | | | | | - |
| | Sig. (2-tailed) | | | | | | | | | | | - |

** Correlation is significant at the .01 level (2-tailed); * Correlation is significant at the .05 level (2-tailed). gray shading indicates that these correlations were computed using the Pearson correlation coefficien

*Group differences at pretest (baseline differences):* Non-parametric data was analysed using the Kruskal-Wallis test, parametric data was analysed with one-way analyses of variance (ANOVA). All results are displayed in Table 14. There were significant base-line group differences in two non-parametric measures, digit span forward and digit span total score. For those two measures, post hoc tests were conducted to identify which of the groups actually differ. Mann-Whitney tests were used for this in combination with a Bonferroni correction to avoid an inflated Type I error rate (Field, 2005). Therefore, the critical level of significance used here was .05 divided by three, or .0167.

For digit span forward, there was a significant difference between the cognitive training and the eccentric training group ($U$= 26.5, $r$= -.58, $p$= .005), but not between cognitive and conventional strength training or eccentric training and conventional strength training (both ps > .0167). The mean score of the cognitive training group was significantly lower at pretest than the mean score of the eccentric training group. Similarly, for the digit span total score, it is again the cognitive training group and the eccentric training group that differ significantly at pretest ($U$= 25.5, $r$= -.56, $p$= .006). There were no other significant differences (all other $p$s > .0167). In the measures which were tested with parametric methods, there was one measure, namely Dual Task Hits, in which there was a significant base-line difference between groups ($F(2, 35) = 3.567$, $p = 039$). However, post hoc tests that used the Bonferroni correction failed to find a significant group difference between any two of the groups. The significant baseline differences will be taken into account when testing the hypotheses by calculating analyses of covariance (ANCOVAs) with the posttest values as dependent variables and the baseline performance scores as covariates.

*Table 14: Group differences at pretest*

| Variable | Cognitive Training M | SD | Conven. Strength Training M | SD | Eccentric strength training M | SD | Kruskal-Wallis H | p |
|---|---|---|---|---|---|---|---|---|
| n | 13 | | 14 | | 11 | | | |
| DS forw | | | | | | | | |
| Pretest | 5.38 | 0.77 | 5.79 | 1.05 | 6.36 | 0.67 | 7.31 | .026*[1] |
| DS back | | | | | | | | |
| Pretest | 4.23 | 1.09 | 4.57 | 1.40 | 4.82 | 0.75 | 1.91 | .384 |
| DS total | | | | | | | | |
| Pretest | 9.62 | 1.33 | 10.36 | 2.06 | 11.18 | 1.08 | 6.97 | .031*[1] |
| Stroop inh. | | | | | | | | |
| Pretest | 29.62 | 12.84 | 22.43 | 7.50 | 20.45 | 6.47 | 5.15 | .076 |
| Free Recall | | | | | | | | |
| Pretest | 6.15 | 2.73 | 5.64 | 4.81 | 5.27 | 2.72 | 1.65 | .438 |

[1] cognitive training < eccentric training

| Variable | Cognitive Training M | SD | Conven. Strength Training M | SD | Eccentric strength training M | SD | F | p |
|---|---|---|---|---|---|---|---|---|
| n | 13 | | 14 | | 11 | | | |
| DST | | | | | | | | |
| Pretest | 36.69 | 8.19 | 37.00 | 7.08 | 36.73 | 8.32 | .006 | .994 |
| WMS | | | | | | | | |
| Pretest | 10.23 | 3.42 | 9.07 | 3.81 | 10.55 | 4.13 | .547 | .584 |
| RT | | | | | | | | |
| Pretest | 0.41 | 0.02 | 0.41 | 0.06 | 0.44 | 0.08 | 1.383 | .264 |
| Dual task hits | | | | | | | | |
| Pretest | 75.90 | 13.71 | 77.49 | 10.31 | 87.11 | 7.66 | 3.567 | .039*[2] |
| Dual task RT | | | | | | | | |
| Pretest | 0.46 | 0.09 | 0.48 | 0.09 | 0.48 | 0.08 | .189 | .829 |
| Recognition | | | | | | | | |
| Pretest | 11.54 | 2.63 | 12.07 | 2.95 | 9.73 | 3.23 | 2.096 | .138 |

[2] post hoc tests failed to find significant differences between groups

*Group differences, changes over time and group\*time interactions*

To give the reader an overview over data, repeated measures analyses of variance were computed with all variables (Table 15). The results from these analyses are as follows: There are significant group effects for digit span forward, digit span total, and Dual task hit scores. All of these variables yielded significant baseline differences between groups, which persisted over time. There is one significant effect of time and one significant interaction effect, both in the Stroop task. These effects will be examined in more difference in the hypothesis testing part, under "hypotheses comparing the effects of the different types of training". There were no other significant effects.

*Table 15: Summary of repeated measures analyses of variance for cognitive measures*

| Variable | | | F | Sig. |
|---|---|---|---|---|
| Speed | Digit Symbol Test | group effect | .150 | .862 |
| | | session effect | 3.428 | .073 |
| | | group*session | .675 | .516 |
| | Reaction Time | group effect | .406 | .670 |
| | | session effect | .085 | .772 |
| | | group*session | .921 | .408 |
| Memory | Digit Span forward | group effect | 5.621 | .008* |
| | | session effect | .114 | .737 |
| | | group*session | 1.128 | .335 |
| | digit Span backward | group effect | 1.132 | .334 |
| | | session effect | .287 | .595 |
| | | group*session | .029 | .972 |
| | Digit Span total | group effect | 4.244 | .022* |
| | | session effect | .440 | .512 |
| | | group*session | .536 | .590 |
| | Wechsler Memory Story | group effect | 1.110 | .341 |
| | | session effect | 2.504 | .123 |
| | | group*session | .434 | .651 |
| | Free Recall | group effect | .575 | .568 |
| | | session effect | 3.584 | .067 |
| | | group*session | .419 | .661 |
| | Recognition | group effect | 2.130 | .134 |
| | | session effect | 1.903 | .177 |
| | | group*session | 1.165 | .324 |
| Executive Functions | Stroop | group effect | 1.974 | .154 |
| | | session effect | 5.531 | .024* |
| | | group*session | 4.024 | .027* |
| | Dual Task Hits | group effect | 3.340 | .047* |
| | | session effect | 2.029 | .163 |
| | | group*session | .109 | .897 |
| | Dual Task Reaction time | group effect | .234 | .792 |
| | | session effect | .437 | .513 |
| | | group*session | 2.377 | .108 |

Note: There were significant basline group differences in Digit Span and Dual Task Hits, which persisted over time.

### 5.1.2 Hypothesis testing

> **Hypotheses regarding eccentric training:** The eccentric training intervention leads to an improvement in speed und executive functions, but not in memory.

For the eccentric training group, parametric analyses were used for Digit Symbol Test (DST), reaction time (RT), Stroop (Strp), Dual Task reaction time($DT_{rt}$), and Wechsler Memory Story (WMS) (Shapiro-Wilks, all $ps > .05$). Dual task hits ($DT_{hits}$), Digit Span, Free Recall and Recognition were tested with non-parametric methods, namely the Wilcoxon Signed Ranks Test. All effect sizes ($r$) were computed according to Field (2005).

Both speed measures failed to yield a significant pre-posttest difference (DST: $M_{pre}= 36.73$, $SE_{pre}= 8.32$, $M_{post}= 37.55$, $SE_{post} = 5.94$, $t(10)= -.655$, $p= .26$ (one-sided), $r= .20$; RT: $M_{pre}= .44$, $SE_{pre}= .08$, $M_{post}= .42$, $SE_{post} = .06$, $t(10)= 1.617$, $p= .07$. (one-sided), $r= .46$). However, it is important to note that the effect for the Reaction time is actually a medium to large effect ($r= .46$). Seeing that the effect is also in the right direction, i.e. the eccentric training group decreased their reaction time in the mean, it is likely that here the statistical power was too low due to the very small sample size ($n=11$) to detect the effect (post hoc power calculations yielded that power was .27; to detect the effect with a power of .80, 120 persons would have been necessary). However, with the present sample size, the first part of the hypothesis cannot be confirmed.

All three measures of executive function also failed to yield a significant pre-posttest difference (Strp: $M_{pre}= 20.45$, $SE_{pre}= 6.47$, $M_{post}= 22.20$, $SE_{post} = 6.45$, $t(10)= -1.268$, $p= .12$ (one-sided), $r= .37$; $DT_{rt}$: $M_{pre}= .48$, $SE_{pre}= .08$, $M_{post}= .46$, $SE_{post} = .06$, $t(10)= .813$, $p= .22$ (one-sided), $r= .25$; $DT_{hits}$ : $Mdn_{pre}= 89.55$, $Mdn_{post}= 92.21$, $z= -.889$, $p= .19$ (one-tailed, $r= -.19$). Even though the effect in the Stroop test is of medium size (according to Field, 2005), it is in the wrong direction (participants actually needed more time at posttest to inhibit the automatic reading reaction); therefore, the hypothesis cannot be confirmed for any of the executive measures.

Memory measures: None of the memory variables yielded a significant pre-post-difference (Digit Span forward: $Mdn_{pre}= 6.00$, $Mdn_{post}= 6.00$, $z= -1.134$, $p= .13$ (one-tailed, $r= -.24$); Digit Span backward: $Mdn_{pre}= 5.00$, $Mdn_{post}= 4.00$, $z= -.575$, $p= .33$ (one-tailed, $r= -.12$); Digit Span total: $Mdn_{pre}= 11.00$,

Mdn$_{post}$= 11.00, $z$= -1.063, $p$= .14 (one-tailed, $r$= -.23); Free Recall: Mdn$_{pre}$= 6.00, Mdn$_{post}$= 6.00, $z$= -.542, $p$= .29 (one-tailed, $r$= -.12); Recognition: Mdn$_{pre}$= 10.00, Mdn$_{post}$= 10.00, $z$= -.462, $p$= .32 (one-tailed, $r$= -.10); Wechsler Memory Story: M$_{pre}$= 10.55, SE$_{pre}$= 4.13, M$_{post}$= 10.27, SE$_{post}$ = 2.24, $t$ (10)= .185, $p$= .86 (one-sided)).

In sum, there is no evidence that eccentric training leads to an improvement in executive functions. For the speed measures, there is also no significant result; however, the effect size is quite large in one case, therefore, it is likely that there was no significant result due to a lack of statistical power. As predicted, there were no significant pre-posttest differences in any memory measures. In short, eccentric training did not lead to an improvement in executive functions and memory; it is possible that it could lead to an improvement in speed, however, with the present sample, the effects do not reach significance.

**Hypotheses regarding conventional strength training:** The conventional strength training intervention leads to an improvement in executive functions und memory, but not in speed.

Neither of the executive measures tested with non-parametric methods yielded a significant pre-posttest difference (DualTask$_{hits}$: Mdn$_{pre}$= 75.36, Mdn$_{post}$= 87.05, $z$= -1.224, $p$= .11 (one-sided), $r$= -.23; DualTask$_{rt}$: Mdn$_{pre}$= .47, Mdn$_{post}$= .43, $z$= -.220, $p$= .41 (one-sided), $r$= -.04). However, there was a significant improvement in the Stroop test (M$_{pre}$= 22.43, SE$_{pre}$= 7.50, M$_{post}$= 18.99, SE$_{post}$ = 7.31, $t$ (13)= 2.683, $p$= .01 (one-sided), $r$= .60).
Therefore, the hypothesis can be partially confirmed for the executive measures.

Concerning the memory measures, again none of the non-parametrically tested measures yielded a significant pre-posttest improvement (DigitSpan$_{forward}$: Mdn$_{pre}$= 6.00, Mdn$_{post}$= 6.00, $z$= -.832, $p$= .20 (one-sided), $r$= -.16; DigitSpan$_{backward}$: Mdn$_{pre}$= 4.50, Mdn$_{post}$= 4.00, $z$= -.302, $p$= .38 (one-sided), $r$= -.06; DigitSpan$_{total}$: Mdn$_{pre}$= 10.0, Mdn$_{post}$= 10.0, $z$= -.318, $p$= .38 (one-sided), $r$= -.06; FreeRecall: Mdn$_{pre}$= 4.5, Mdn$_{post}$= 6.0, $z$= -.787, $p$= .22 (one-sided), $r$= -.15).

In the memory measures tested with parametric methods, there was a significant pre-post difference in the Recognition measure (M$_{pre}$= 12.07, SE$_{pre}$= 2.95, M$_{post}$= 9.86, SE$_{post}$ = 3.46, $t$ (13)= 2.060, $p$= .03 (one-sided), $r$= .50). However, as can be seen from the means, this effect a worsening instead of an improvement. In the Wechsler memory story, there was no significant pre-posttest improvement (M$_{pre}$= 9.07, SE$_{pre}$= 3.81, M$_{post}$= 8.07, SE$_{post}$ = 3.43, $t$ (13)= 1.109, $p$= .14 (one-sided), $r$= .29.).

In the speed measures, there was a significant change over time in the Digit Symbol Test (M$_{pre}$= 37.00, SE$_{pre}$= 7.08, M$_{post}$= 39.86, SE$_{post}$ = 2.05, $t$ (13)= -1.881, $p$= .04 (one-sided)), but not in the Reaction time task (Mdn$_{pre}$= .40, Mdn$_{post}$= .42, $z$= -.031, $p$= .49 (one-sided), $r$= .01).

In sum, this hypothesis can be partially confirmed for the executive functions (there was a significant improvement in the Stroop test); however, there is no indication whatsoever that conventional muscle training leads to an improvement in memory. This part of the hypothesis cannot be confirmed. Furthermore, there was an unexpected improvement in one speed task (Digit Symbol Test). The hypothesis as a whole can therefore not be confirmed.

> **Hypotheses regarding cognitive training:** The cognitive training group will show a pre-posttest improvement in memory, speed, and executive functions, even though the tasks used at pre- and posttest were not practiced during the intervention (transfer effects).

In the group of memory measures, only Free Recall and Wechsler Memory Story yielded a significant pre-posttest difference (Free Recall: $Mdn_{pre}$= 6.00, $Mdn_{post}$= 7.00, $z$= -2.177, $p$= .02 (one-sided), $r$= -.43; WMS: $M_{pre}$= 10.23, $SE_{pre}$= 3.41, $M_{post}$= 8.46, $SE_{post}$ = 4.31, $t$ (12)= 1.791, $p$= .05 (one-sided), $r$= .46). However, there was only an improvement in Free Recall; in the Wechsler Story, there was actually a deterioration observed. The other memory measures did not yield significant results ($DigitSpan_{forward}$: $Mdn_{pre}$= 6.00, $Mdn_{post}$= 5.00, $z$= -.447, $p$= .33 (one-sided), $r$= -.09; $DigitSpan_{backward}$: $Mdn_{pre}$= 4.00, $Mdn_{post}$= 4.00, $z$= -.213, $p$= .42 (one-sided), $r$= -.04; $DigitSpan_{total}$: $M_{pre}$= 9.62, $SE_{pre}$= 1.33, $M_{post}$= 9.46, $SE_{post}$ = 1.27, $t$ (12)= .365, $p$= .36 (one-sided), $r$= .15; Recognition: $M_{pre}$= 11.54, $SE_{pre}$= 2.63, $M_{post}$= 11.46, $SE_{post}$ = 3.41, $t$ (12)= .058, $p$= .48 (one-sided), $r$= .02). Therefore, of all memory measures, there was only a significant pre-posttest improvement in Free Recall (Figure 5).

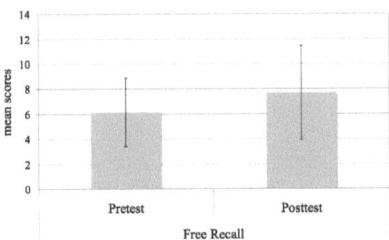

*Figure 5: Improvement in the cognitive training group from pretest to posttest in Free Recall*

In the group of speed measures, there was no significant pre-posttest change in either Digit Symbol Test or Reaction Time task (DST: $M_{pre}$= 36.69, $SE_{pre}$= 8.19, $M_{post}$= 37.62, $SE_{post}$ = 7.02, $t$ (12)= -.654, $p$= .26 (one-sided), $r$= -.19; RT: $M_{pre}$= .41, $SE_{pre}$= .02, $M_{post}$= .42, $SE_{post}$ = .05, $t$ (12)= -1.224, $p$= .12 (one-sided), $r$= -.33).

As for the tests measuring executive aspects, there was a significant improvement in the Stroop test (Mdn$_{pre}$= 29.00, Mdn$_{post}$= 23.00, $z$= -2.062, $p$= .02 (one-sided), $r$= -.40). Participants needed significantly less time at posttest to inhibit the automatic reading reaction than at pretest (see Figure 6). In the two dual taks measures, there were no significant effects (DualTask$_{hits}$: Mdn$_{pre}$= 75.65, Mdn$_{post}$= 81.91, $z$= -.874, $p$= .19 (one-sided), $r$= -.17; DualTask$_{rt}$: M$_{pre}$= .46, SE$_{pre}$= .09, M$_{post}$= .52, SE$_{post}$ = .07, $t$ (12)= -1.675, $p$= .06 (one-sided), $r$= .44).

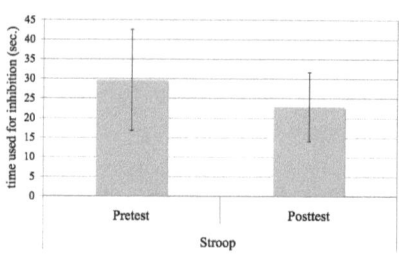

*Figure 6: Improvement in the cognitive training group from pretest to posttest in the Stroop task*

In sum, there was an improvement in Free Recall and Stroop task. These two results can be interpreted as transfer effects (for more on this, please consult the discussion section). However, the hypothesis as a whole cannot be confirmed, as there was no improvement in speed measures.

> **Hypotheses comparing the effects of the different types of training:**
> 1. The improvement in executive functions is smaller in the conventional training group than in the eccentric exercise group.
> 2. The cognitive training group shows the greatest improvement in executive functions of all three training groups.
> 3. Cognitive training is more effective in improving memory performance than either eccentric or conventional strength training.

The first and second hypotheses were tested with repeated measures analyses of variance, followed if indicated by Games-Howell post hoc tests and planned contrasts (Helmert contrasts). The Games-Howell procedure was chosen as it is considered accurate yet powerful when sample sizes are unequal (Field, 2005, p. 341). The analyses are summarized in Table 16.

The results show that there were no significant effects for Dual Task reaction time (interaction session*training group: $F(2, 35) = 2.38$, $p= .108$; main effect group: $F(2, 35) = .234$, $p= .792$). There was also no significant interaction for Dual task hits ($F(2, 35) = .109$, $p= .897$), however, there was a significant main effect for group ($F(2, 35) = 3.340$, $p= .047$), with Games-Howell post hoc tests indicating a significant difference between the eccentric training and conventional strength training group, with the eccentric training group scoring higher at both testing times (Games-Howell p=.037).
There was a significant interaction effect in the Stroop task, $F(2, 35) = 4.024$, $p= .027$, indicating that the scores of three training groups developed differently from pre- to posttest. Looking at Figure 7, it becomes clear that while the time used for inhibiting the inappropriate response decreased in the cognitive and conventional strength training group (i.e. those two groups actually improved), the results of the eccentric training group showed the opposite pattern. Therefore, the first part of the hypothesis can certainly not be confirmed.
Planned contrasts were computed to test the second part of the hypothesis, namely that cognitive training shows the greatest improvement of all training groups. Results of Helmert contrasts show that there is a significant difference between cognitive training and physical training, with cognitive training leading to greater improvement ($p=.029$, one-tailed).

*Table 16: Repeated measures analyses summary of executive measures*

| Source | df | SS | MS | F | Sign. |
|---|---|---|---|---|---|
| **Stroop** | | | | | |
| | | Between subjects | | | |
| exercise group | 2 | 475.137 | 237.568 | 1.974 | .154 |
| Error 1 | 35 | 4212.364 | 120.353 | | |
| | | Within subjects | | | |
| Session | 1 | 149.733 | 149.733 | 5.531 | .024 |
| exercise group*session | 2 | 217.883 | 108.942 | 4.024 | .027 |
| Error 2 | 35 | 947.520 | 27.072 | | |
| **Dual task hits** | | | | | |
| | | Between subjects | | | |
| exercise group | 2 | 1821.879 | 910.940 | 3.340 | .047 |
| Error 1 | 35 | 9545.773 | 272.736 | | |
| | | Within subjects | | | |
| Session | 1 | 149.083 | 149.083 | 2.029 | .163 |
| exercise group*session | 2 | 16.070 | 8.035 | .109 | .897 |
| Error 2 | 35 | 2571.261 | 73.465 | | |
| **Dual Task Reaction Time** | | | | | |
| | | Between subjects | | | |
| exercise group | 2 | .005 | .003 | .234 | .792 |
| Error 1 | 35 | .382 | .011 | | |
| | | Within subjects | | | |
| Session | 1 | .002 | .002 | .437 | .513 |
| exercise group*session | 2 | .022 | .011 | 2.377 | .108 |
| Error 2 | 35 | .161 | .005 | | |

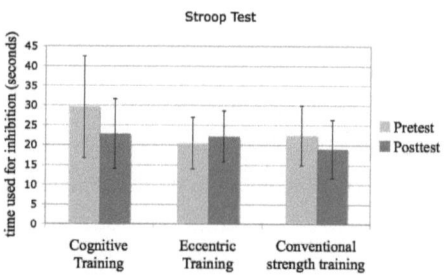

*Figure 7: Change from pre- to posttest in stroop test*

The third hypothesis about whether cognitive training was more successful in improving memory performance was tested with repeated measures analyses of variance for the variables Wechsler memory, Free Recall, and Recognition. This analysis did not yield any significant interaction effects (WMS: $F(2,35)= .434$, $p=.651$ ; Free Recall: $F(2,35)= .419$, $p=.661$, $r= -.15^2$; Recognition: $F(2,35)= 1.165$., $p= .324$) (Table 17), indicating that there was no difference in how the different trainings had influenced the memory scores.

As there were baseline differences between groups in digit span forward, digit span backward and digit span total score, these variables were assessed with an Analysis of Covariance (ANCOVA), followed by planned contrasts where indicated. The posttest scores were entered as dependent variables and the pretest scores as covariates. For all three digit span measures, there was no significant main effect for training group ($DS_{forward}$: $F(2, 34)= 2.795$, $p=.075$; $DS_{backward}$: $F(2, 34)= .313$, $p=.733$; $DS_{total}$: $F(2, 34)= 1.812$, $p=.179$). However, in all three cases the covariate had a significant effect on the posttest scores ($DS_{forward}$: $F(2, 34)= 8.671$, $p=.006$; $DS_{backward}$: $F(2, 34)= 4.263$, $p=.047$; $DS_{total}$: $F(1, 34)= 11.243$, $p= .002$).

In sum, it cannot be confirmed that cognitive training lead to a greater improvement in memory measures than eccentric and conventional strength training. However, it is important to note the magnitude of the standard deviations (see Figure 8); obviously, there was a great degree of variation in the sample. Some people did improve with training, whereas others did not. In view of this, it will be important to examine more closely which persons were able to profit from the trainings and which persons did not. What are the "prerequisites" so a person can benefit from a training program? A first indicator stems from the ANCOVA computed above. It appears as if the baseline performance is an indicator of subsequent improvement. This hypothesis as well as other possibilities will be addressed in more detail in the aposteriori hypotheses.

*Table 17: Summary of repeated measures analyses of variance for memory variables*

| Source | df | SS | MS | F | Sign. |
|---|---|---|---|---|---|
| **Wechsler Memory Story** | | | | | |
| | | Between subjects | | | |
| exercise type | 2 | 41.624 | 20.812 | 1.110 | .341 |
| Error 1 | 35 | 656.060 | 18.745 | | |
| | | Within subjects | | | |
| Session | 1 | 19.338 | 19.338 | 2.504 | .123 |
| exercise type*session | 2 | 6.703 | 3.351 | .434 | .651 |
| Error 2 | 35 | 270.245 | 7.721 | | |

---

[2] $r$ was chosen here as effect size rather than $\omega$, as $\omega$ cannot be used when the sample sizes are unequal.

| Free Recall | | | | | |
|---|---|---|---|---|---|
| | Between subjects | | | | |
| exercise type | 2 | 25.902 | 12.951 | .575 | .568 |
| Error 1 | 35 | 787.729 | 22.507 | | |
| | Within subjects | | | | |
| Session | 1 | 17.600 | 17.600 | 3.584 | .067 |
| exercise type*session | 2 | 4.112 | 2.056 | .419 | .661 |
| Error 2 | 35 | 171.888 | 4.911 | | |
| **Recognition** | | | | | |
| | Between subjects | | | | |
| exercise type | 2 | 47.818 | 23.909 | 2.130 | .134 |
| Error 1 | 35 | 392.919 | 11.226 | | |
| | Within subjects | | | | |
| Session | 1 | 14.729 | 14.729 | 1.903 | .177 |
| exercise type*session | 2 | 18.035 | 9.017 | 1.165 | .324 |
| Error 2 | 35 | 270.913 | 7.740 | | |

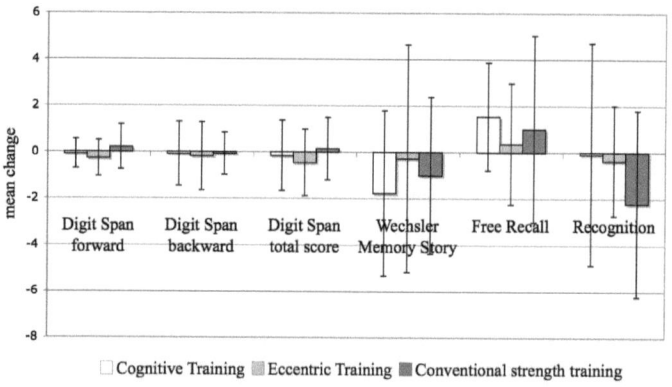

*Figure 8: Mean change scores of memory measures*

**Further question of interest:**
Are age, IQ, gender, or baseline performance associated with subsequent improvement or decline?

What distinguishes persons who profit from an intervention from persons who do not? Clearly, there some people in the ExTrA study who improved tremendously over time, whereas others remained stable or even deteriorated (for an example, see the scatterplots in Figure 9). It is of great scientific and practical interest to find out what differentiates "successful" and "unsuccessful" participants. There are several possibilities: For one, it could be that the younger participants improved more than the older ones. Another alternative would be that the IQ is predicitive for the extent of pre-posttest improvement, or that there is a gender effect. Last but not least, it has been postulated that participants with a low performance level at pretest tend to profit more from training than do participants who had an already high performance level. All these possibilities will be examined in turn.

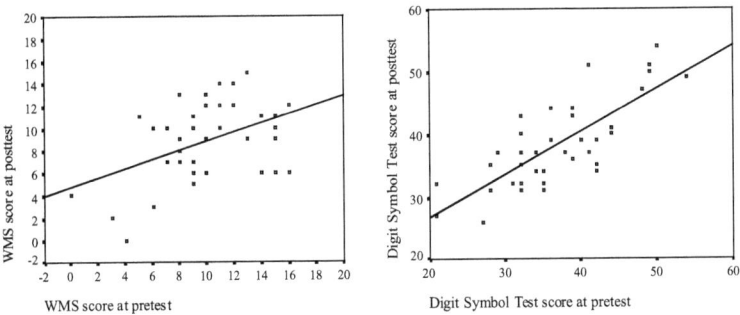

*Figure 9: Pretest scores in relation to posttest scores (WMS, Digit Span total)*

To examine whether age was associated with subsequent improvement, one-tailed correlations were computed between age and all pre-post-difference values. None of these correlations reached statistical significance (all ps > .05). Second, from the total sample of participants, two extreme groups in terms of age were extracted. The cut-off was calculated by adding respectively subtracting one standard deviation from the mean age. The "young old" therefore were defined as being younger than 78 years (six participants), and the "old old" group was defined as being at least 85 years old (seven participants). The pre-posttest difference scores of these two groups were then compared with the Mann-Whitney test. There was only one measure which yielded a significant pre-posttest difference between the "young old" and the "old old" of our sample, Free Recall ($Mdn_{young\ old}$ = 3.5, $Mdn_{old\ old}$ = 0.0, $U$ = 8.00, $p$ = .04 (one-tailed), $r$ = .52). All other results did not reach statistical significance (all $ps$ > .05). Therefore it cannot be generally confirmed that younger participants show a greater pre-posttest improvement than older participants.

However, it would be possible that participants with higher IQs profited more from the trainings than participants with lower IQs. To test this theory, correlations were calculated between MWT-A pretest scores as indicator of IQ and pre-posttest difference scores. None of these correlations reached statistical significance. Furthermore, as the variance in MWT-A scores was very low ($M$=31.97, $SD$=2.35) there were not enough extreme cases to calculate extreme group comparisons. A high IQ therefore does not seem to be associated with greater profit.

To test whether men and women differed in their rate of pre-posttest improvement, Mann-Whitney U-tests and independent t-tests were conducted, depending on whether the variables were normally distributed. However, there were no significant differences in improvement between men and women (all $ps$ > .05; Men and women also did not differ in their performance at pretest, with one exception, Dual Task reaction time ($M_{men}$ = .43, $SD_{men}$ = .07, $M_{women}$ = .49, $SD_{women}$ = .09, $t(36)$= -2.191, $p$= .04 two-tailed), in which men reacted significantly faster than women). The same calculations were repeated for each training group separately, with the same result. It needs to be mentioned though that the sample size in these calculations was so small that an effect would have had to be extremely big to be detected. As this is rarely the case in gender differences, the non-significant result is not surprising.

The last question concerned the issue whether a high baseline performance level tends to be associated with subsequent decline while low baseline scores tend to be associated with subsequent improvement in the same task ("regression to the mean"). This question was examined by calculating correlations between baseline performance and subsequent change for different cognitive measures (for memory, executive function and speed / reaction time measures).

*Memory measures:* With the exception of Free recall, all memory measure baseline scores (i.e. digit span forward, digit span backward, digit span total score, Wechsler memory story, and recognition) correlated significantly with the subsequent change in performance to posttest (Spearman's rho, all $\rho$ < .001, see Table 18).

*Speed:* Both measures used to assess psychomotor speed in this thesis, Digit Symbol Test and Reaction time task, showed significant correlations between baseline scores and subsequent change (Digit Symbol Test: $\rho$ =-.478, $p$< .002; Reaction time: $\rho$ =-.547, $p$< .000). Both correlations were in the direction that the performance of people who started out with a high baseline level tended to deteriorate, whereas people with a low baseline level tended to improve (Figure 10; please take note that the Digit Symbol test assesses speed by measuring the number of items completed within a certain time limit, whereas the Reaction time task assesses reaction time. Therefore, a negative change value indicates deterioration in the Digit Symbol Test and improvement in the Reaction time task, and vice versa).

*Table 18: Correlations between baseline memory performance and subsequent change*

| baseline scores | | Digit Span forward | Digit Span backward | change (difference pretest-posttest) Digit Span total | WMS | Recognition | Free Recall |
|---|---|---|---|---|---|---|---|
| Digit Span forward | Rho Sig. (2-tailed) | -.678*** .000 | | | | | |
| Digit Span backward | Rho Sig. (2-tailed) | | -.717*** .000 | | | | |
| Digit Span total | Rho Sig. (2-tailed) | | | -.683*** .000 | | | |
| WMS | Rho Sig. (2-tailed) | | | | -.527*** .001 | | |
| recognition | Rho Sig. (2-tailed) | | | | | -.639*** .000 | |
| Free Recall | Rho Sig. (2-tailed) | | | | | | -.234 .158 |

\*\*\* Correlation is significant at the .001 level (2-tailed).

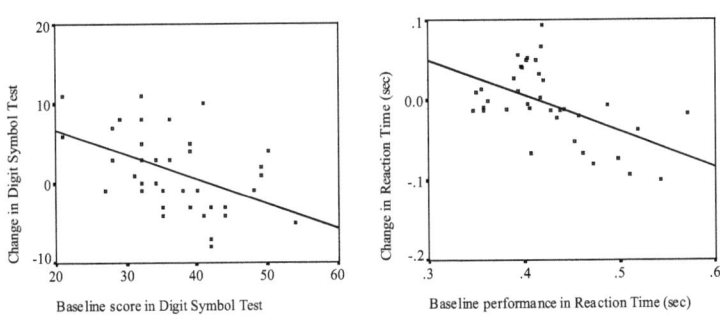

*Figure 10: Digit Symbol Test and Reaction time baseline scores in relation to subsequent change*

*Executive functions:* The baseline performance in the Stroop test correlated significantly with subsequent change, $\rho=-.526$, $p<.001$. Dual task hits baseline performance was not significantly correlated with subsequent change, $\rho=-.287$, $p=.081$. The baseline performance in Dual Task reaction time was significantly correlated with subsequent change, $\rho=-.322$, $p=.048$; however, a look at the scatterplot (Figure 11) reveals that this correlation is an artefact caused by one point of data, which lies more than two standard deviations away from the mean score ($M=.01$, $SD=.10$, datapoint at .41). In view of this, the correlation was repeated without the outlier. This correlation does not reach statistical significance anymore ($\rho=-.266$, $p=.112$, see Figure 11).

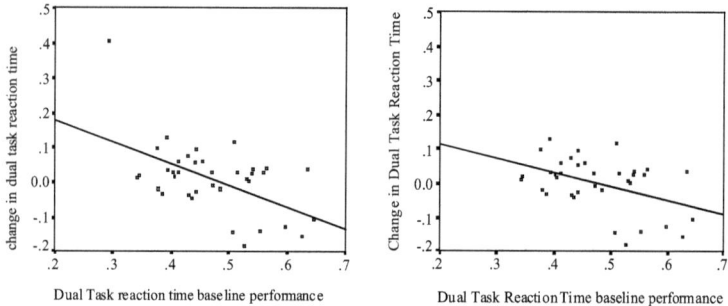

*Figure 11: Correlation between Dualtask baseline performance and subsequent change (left with outlier included, right without outlier)*

In conclusion, for all memory measures except Free Recall, the theory that a high baseline performance level tends to be associated with subsequent decline while low baseline scores tend to be associated with subsequent improvement can be confirmed. It can also be confirmed for the speed / reaction time measures. Things are less clear where executive function measures are concerned. While the theory can be confirmed for the Stroop task, it cannot be confirmed for the two Dual Task measures. It therefore appears that there is a regression to the mean in a majority of the measures examined.

### 5.1.3 Summary of cognitive results

None of the physical trainings had an effect on memory. While this was expected for eccentric training, it had been hypothesized that conventional strength training might also lead to an improvement in memory due to the results of another study with resistance exercise (Perrig-Chiello et al., 1998).

However, there was no indication whatsoever in our study that conventional strength training might enhance memory. The cognitive training group showed an improvement in visual long-term memory, but not in memory span, working memory or long term verbal memory.

With regard to executive functions, conventional strength training and cognitive training both led to an improvement in inhibition. There was no improvement in task coordination assessed by dual task measures. Against expectation, eccentric training did not lead to an improvement in any of the executive function measures. It appears that the dual-task characteristic of adjusting one's use of strength according to the feedback on a computer screen does not transfer to other dual tasks.

Concerning the measures of speed, only the conventional strength training group showed a significant improvement (in Digit Symbol Test). In the eccentric training group, there was a medium to large effect (in Reaction Time), which failed to reach significance, probably due to the small sample size. The cognitive training did not appear to affect any speed measures.

What was striking in almost all measures was the great variance of results. Some participants improved quite impressively, whereas others deteriorated. Additional analyses yielded that neither age, gender nor intelligence were related to amount of improvement. However, baseline performance was indicative of subsequent improvement or decline. It therefore appears that "those who have a lot also have a lot to lose".

## 5.2 Well-being

### 5.2.1 Descriptives, distribution testing, correlations

*Descriptives*: Means and standard deviations of the well-being measures are shown in Table 19. It is important to note that all of these values obtained in our study are very high in comparison to the norm values for 76-85 year olds (means of the norm sample ranging from 60.18 in physical well-being to 67.30 in the environment subscale; Angermeyer et al., 2000).

*Table 19: Means and standard deviations of the WHOQOL-BREF domains*

|  | Cognitive training n=13 | | | | Eccentric training n=11 | | | | Strength training n=14 | | | |
|---|---|---|---|---|---|---|---|---|---|---|---|---|
|  | pretest | | posttest | | pretest | | posttest | | pretest | | posttest | |
|  | M | SD | M | SD | M | SD | M | SD | M | SD | M | SD |
| **WHOQOL** | | | | | | | | | | | | |
| Physical | 68.46 | 2.17 | 76.65 | 10.78 | 76.19 | 2.96 | 85.60 | 12.14 | 73.61 | 1.73 | 83.42 | 7.75 |
| Psychol. | 76.60 | 2.73 | 77.24 | 7.14 | 75.00 | 2.64 | 77.27 | 7.54 | 75.89 | 1.76 | 79.46 | 4.16 |
| Social | 83.33 | 4.32 | 78.21 | 8.70 | 84.09 | 4.12 | 77.27 | 11.84 | 72.62 | 2.54 | 79.76 | 9.65 |
| Environm. | 91.11 | 1.49 | 91.83 | 5.92 | 90.06 | 1.73 | 94.03 | 5.49 | 90.18 | 1.60 | 92.41 | 6.57 |
| global | 82.69 | 3.33 | 87.50 | 11.41 | 85.23 | 3.29 | 89.77 | 10.92 | 83.04 | 3.10 | 87.50 | 10.96 |
| total | 402.2 | 30.56 | 411.4 | 29.27 | 410.6 | 35.82 | 423.4 | 31.33 | 395.3 | 26.53 | 422.6 | 23.67 |

Note: each domain of the WHOQOL has a range of 0-100.

*Distribution testing*: Skewness and kurtosis of WHOQOL-Bref pretest and posttest scores were within acceptable range (i.e. below 2.58, as recommended by Field, 2005, for small samples). In the full sample (i.e. not divided into training groups), the domains social, environment and global deviated significantly from normal distribution at pretest (Shapiro-Wilks, all $ps < .05$). At posttest, all domains except physical well-being violated the assumption of normal distribution (Shapiro-Wilks, all $ps < .05$). Therefore, non-parametric analyses were used for all WHOQOL-domains except physical well-being, which was analysed with parametric methods. The sum of all domains was normally distributed and therefore tested with parametric methods. As for the pre-post difference values, only physical and environmental well-being as well as the sum of all domains (WHOQOL_tot) were normally distributed in the full sample, and thus tested with parametric methods.

*Pre-post correlations*: Spearman's rho was used to compute correlations, as the data set is small and did not conform to parametric standards. Each of the WHOQOL-Bref domains showed a significant pre-post correlation with itself (all $\rho > .55$, all $p$s $< .00$), confirming retest-reliability. Furthermore, physical well-being at pre-test correlated with psychological ($\rho = .52$, $p < .00$) and global well-being at posttest ($\rho = .35$, $p < .03$); psychological well-being at pretest correlated significantly with physical well-being at posttest ($\rho = .33$, $p < .04$), and global well-being at pretest correlated significantly with physical well-being at posttest ($\rho = .33$, $p < .04$). There were no other significant pre-posttest correlations (Table 20).

*Table 20: Pre-posttest correlations of the WHOQOL domains*

| | | Posttest | | | | |
|---|---|---|---|---|---|---|
| | | Physical | Psychol. | Social | Environm. | global |
| **Pretest** | | | | | | |
| Physical | rho | .667*** | .520** | .032 | .205 | .354* |
| | Sign. | .000 | .001 | .847 | .217 | .029 |
| Psychol. | rho | .329* | .602*** | .022 | .213 | .201 |
| | Sign. | .044 | .000 | .895 | .200 | .227 |
| Social | rho | .018 | .152 | .554*** | .021 | .159 |
| | Sign. | .915 | .362 | .000 | .899 | .339 |
| Environm. | rho | .125 | .071 | -.021 | .564*** | .193 |
| | Sign. | .455 | .670 | .901 | .000 | .245 |
| global | rho | .333* | .268 | .061 | .295 | .609*** |
| | Sign. | .041 | .104 | .716 | .072 | .000 |

\* $p < .05$, \*\* $p < .01$, \*\*\* $p < .001$

*Pre-post effects in the full sample:*
The domains physical, psychological, environmental and global well-being all showed significant pre-post differences. Scores of the psychological domain at pretest ($Mdn$=77.08) were significantly lower than at posttest ($Mdn$=79.17, $z$=-1.96, $p$= .05, $r$= -.22). The pattern was basically the same for the „environment"-domain, with pretest scores ($Mdn$=90.63) being significantly lower than posttest scores ($Mdn$=93.75, $z$=-2.40, $p$= .016, $r$=-.28). For the social well-being domain, pretest scores ($Mdn$=83.33, $M$=79.61) did not differ significantly from posttest scores ($Mdn$=75.00, $M$=78.51, $z$=-.724, $p$= .47). In the global well-being domain, pretest scores ($Mdn$=81.25) were again significantly lower than posttest scores ($Mdn$=87.5, $z$=-2.56, $p$= .01, $r$= -.29).

*Group differences at pre-test (baseline differences)*
As the groups were not perfectly parallelized in terms of age, health, and education variables, it is crucial to assess whether there were group differences in the dependent variables from the outset. In the WHO-QOL Bref, there was a significant group difference in the social domain, with participants in the strength training condition scoring significantly lower than participants in the cognitive and eccentric training groups ($M_{strength}$=72.62, $M_{cognitive}$=83.33, $M_{eccentric}$=84.09, Kruskal-Wallis $H(2)$=6.91, $p$= .03). There were no other significant a priori differences between groups.

*Effects of group, effects of session and group\*session interactions*
To give the reader a better idea of the data, Table 21 presents a summary of repated measures regression analyses computed for all WHOQOL-Bref scores. There were several significant effects: The domains physical, environment, global as well as the total score yielded significant session effects, with significantly higher scores at posttest than at pretest. There was also a significant group\*session interaction in the social domain. Whereas in the conventional strength training group there was an improvement in the social domain from pre- to posttest, the cognitive and eccentric training groups showed the opposite pattern.

*Table 21: Repeated measures analyses summary for WHOQOL-Bref*

| Source | | F | Sig. |
|---|---|---|---|
| WHOQOL-Bref physical domain | group effect | 3.124 | .056 |
| | session effect | 50.676 | .000* |
| | group*session | .151 | .860 |
| WHOQOL-Bref psychological domain | group effect | .175 | .840 |
| | session effect | 3.218 | .081 |
| | group*session | .531 | .593 |
| WHOQOL-Bref social domain | group effect | .833 | .443 |
| | session effect | .927 | .342 |
| | group*session | 7.315 | .002* |
| WHOQOL-Bref environmental domain | group effect | .066 | .936 |
| | session effect | 7.242 | .011* |
| | group*session | 1.140 | .332 |
| WHOQOL-Bref global domain | group effect | .204 | .816 |
| | session effect | 7.827 | .008* |
| | group*session | .004 | .996 |
| WHOQOL-Bref total score | group effect | .479 | .623 |
| | session effect | 15.694 | .000* |
| | group*session | 1.883 | .167 |

*Correlations between cognitive and well-being measures at pretest*

There are almost no significant correlations between cognitive and well-being measures at pretest (Table 22). Only four correlations reach significance. Digit Span forwards correlates significantly with the WHOQOL-psychological subscale ($\rho = -.430$, $p= .007$), as does Dual Task reaction time ($r = -.401$, $p= .013$), and Wechsler memory correlates significantly with the WHOQOL global subscale ($\rho= .417$, $p=.009$). Wechsler memory also correlated significantly with the overall score of well-being ($\rho= .378$, $p=.019$). There were no other significant correlations (all $ps > .05$).

*Table 22: Correlations between WHOQOL-BREF domains and cognitive measures at pretest*

| | | Physical well-being | Psychol. well-being | Social well-being | environment | global well-being | well-being overall |
|---|---|---|---|---|---|---|---|
| Digit Span forward | Rho | -.187 | -.430** | -.009 | -.040 | -.159 | -.229 |
| | Sig. (2-tailed) | .260 | .007 | .959 | .812 | .342 | .168 |
| Digit Span backward | Rho | .242 | .272 | .018 | .032 | .232 | .215 |
| | Sig. (2-tailed) | .144 | .098 | .912 | .848 | .161 | .194 |
| Digit Span total | Rho | .033 | -.069 | .011 | .030 | .019 | -.016 |
| | Sig. (2-tailed) | .842 | .680 | .948 | .858 | .911 | .926 |
| Stroop inhibition | Rho | -.106 | .062 | .131 | .058 | .027 | .058 |
| | Sig. (2-tailed) | .528 | .711 | .434 | .728 | .872 | .729 |
| cgft - Reaction | Rho | -.046 | -.072 | -.008 | -.179 | -.039 | -.112 |
| | Sig. (2-tailed) | .783 | .667 | .963 | .281 | .816 | .505 |
| cgft - Recogn. | Rho | -.146 | -.160 | -.010 | .023 | -.042 | -.038 |
| | Sig. (2-tailed) | .383 | .336 | .953 | .891 | .802 | .819 |
| cgft - Free Recall | Rho | .005 | .007 | .305 | .069 | -.003 | .095 |
| | Sig. (2-tailed) | .978 | .966 | .062 | .682 | .987 | .570 |
| Dual Task hits | Rho | -.007 | -.197 | -.014 | -.223 | -.015 | -.133 |
| | Sig. (2-tailed) | .967 | .237 | .933 | .179 | .929 | .425 |
| Digit Symbol Test | Rho | .170 | .123 | .095 | .007 | .151 | .201 |
| | Sig. (2-tailed) | .307 | .462 | .572 | .965 | .364 | .226 |
| Wechsler Memory | Rho | .308 | .157 | .242 | .053 | .417** | .378* |
| | Sig. (2-tailed) | .060 | .346 | .144 | .753 | .009 | .019 |
| Dual task RT | Rho | -.205 | -.401* | -.095 | -.089 | -.135 | -.272 |
| | Sig. (2-tailed) | .217 | .013 | .572 | .597 | .420 | .098 |

** Correlation is significant at the .01 level (2-tailed)., * Correlation is significant at the .05 level (2-tailed). Gray shading indicates that these correlations were computed using the Pearson correlation.

### 5.2.2 Hypothesis testing

> **Physical training hypotheses**: Physical training leads to an increase in overall well-being. Furthermore, on the domain level, physical training leads to an improvement in physical and psychological well-being. However, the improvement is greater in physical well-being.

To test whether physical training leads to an increase in overall well-being, the eccentric and the conventional strength training group were analyzed together as one group, with a paired samples t-test. The result confirms a significant increase in well-being over time, $M_{pre}= 402.04$, $SE_{pre}= 31.23$, $M_{post}= 422.93$, $SE_{post}=26.29$, $t(24)=-4.242$, $p= .000$ one-sided, $r= .65$. Similarly, there was also a significant improvement over time in the physical and psychological domains (physical domain: $M_{pre}=74.74$, $SE_{pre}=1.61$, $M_{post}=84.12$, $SE_{post}= 9.73$, $t(24)=-6.379$, $p= .000$ one-sided, $r= .79$; psychological domain: $M_{pre}=75.50$, $SE_{pre}= 1.49$, $M_{post}=78.50$, $SE_{post}= 1.17$, $t(24)=-2.753$, $p= .006$ one-sided, $r= .49$).

When examining the two training groups separately, starting with the eccentric training group, there were significant pre-post differences observed for the physical domain (parametric calculation). Physical well-being was significantly lower at pre- than at posttest ($M_{pre}=76.19$, $SE_{pre}=9.82$, $M_{post}=85.09$, $SE_{post}=12.14$, $t(10)=-3.617$, $p= .004$ one-sided, $r= .75$). The psychological domain did not show any significant changes over time ($M_{pre}= 75.00$, $SE_{pre}= 8.74$, $M_{post}= 77.27$, $SE_{post}= 7.53$, $p> .05$) (see Figure 12). There was a medium sized effect in overall well-being; however, this effect did not reach statistical significance ($M_{pre}=410.57$, $SD_{pre}=35.82$, $M_{post}=423.42$, $SD_{post}=31.33$, $t(10)=-1.645$, $p= .07$ one-sided, $r= .50$). In the conventional strength training group, there were significant pre-posttest differences in overall well-being ($M_{pre}=395.34$, $SD_{pre}=26.53$, $M_{post}=422.56$, $SD_{post}=23.67$, $t(13)=-4.996$, $p= .000$, $r= .81$), as well as in the physical and psychological domain (Figure 12). Physical well-being was significantly lower at pre- than at posttest ($M_{pre}=73.61$, $SE_{pre}=6.49$, $M_{post}=83.42$, $SE_{post}=7.75$, $t(13)=-5.208$, $p= .000$, $r= .95$). A significant increase was also found for psychological well-being ($Mdn_{pre}=79.17$, $Mdn_{post}=79.17$; $M_{pre}=75.89$, $M_{post}=79.46$, $z=-2.02$, $p= .022$ one-sided, $r=- .38$).

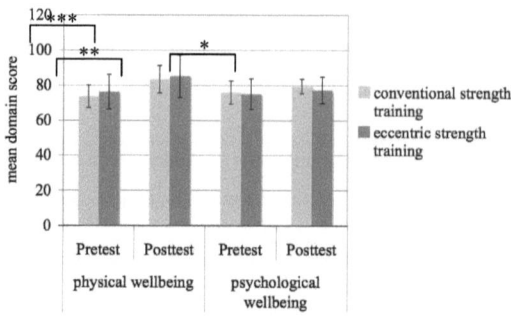

*Figure 12: Pre- and posttest scores in two domains of well-being for the physical training groups*


A Wilcoxon signed-rank test was used to test the hypothesis that the improvement was greater in the physical than in the psychological domain, as the same participants completed both the physical and the psychological domain questions. As could already be gathered from the preliminary analyses, in the eccentric training group the improvement in the physical domain was significantly greater than the improvement in the psychological domain (seeing as there was no significant improvement at all), $Mdn_{phys}$= 6.25, $Mdn_{psych}$= 0.00; $M_{phys}$= 8.87, $M_{psych}$= 2.27, $z$= -2.401, $p$= .008 one-sided, $r$= -.51.

Therefore, the hypothesis can be confirmed for the eccentric training group. For the conventional muscle training group, the improvement in physical well-being was also greater than the improvement in psychological well-being, $Mdn_{phys}$= 11.55, $Mdn_{psych}$= 4.17; $M_{phys}$= 9.81, $M_{psych}$= 3.57, $z$= -2.983, $p$= .002 one-sided, $r$= -.56. When both groups are analyzed together, this result is confirmed ($z$= -3.727, $p$= .000).

Therefore, this hypothesis can be confirmed in its entirety.

**Cognitive training hypotheses**: Cognitive training leads to an increase in both physical and psychological well-being. However, the increase in psychological well-being is expected to be greater than the one in physical well-being.

The first part of the hypothesis was tested with paired samples t-tests. Results for the physical domain showed a significant improvement from pre- to posttest ($M_{pre}$= 86.46, $SE_{pre}$= 7.83, $M_{post}$= 76.65, $SE_{post}$=10.78, $t(12)$=-3.644, $p$= .002 one-sided, $r$= .72). The test for the psychological domain failed to reach significance ($M_{pre}$= 76.60, $SE_{pre}$= 9.85, $M_{post}$= 77.24, $SE_{post}$=7.14, $t(12)$=-.230, $p$= .411 one-sided, $r$= .07).

The second part of the hypothesis was tested with a paired samples t-test which compared the improvement scores. This yielded indeed a significant difference between the improvement in physical and psychological well-being; however, as was already to be expected from the first part of the hypothesis, the difference is in the wrong direction ($M_{physdif}$= 8.18, $SE_{physdif}$= 8.10, $M_{psydif}$= .64, $SE_{psydif}$= 10.04, $t(12)$= 2.301, $p$= .020. one-sided, $r$= .55; see Figure 13) The improvement in physical well-being was much greater than in psychological well-being. Therefore, this hypothesis cannot be confirmed.

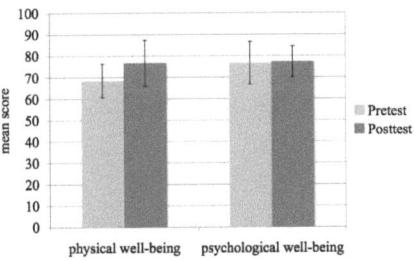

*Figure 13: Pre-posttest effects in the physical and psychological domains for the cognitive training group*

**Hypotheses concerned with training comparisons:**
1. Both physical training as well as cognitive training leads to an improvement in overall well-being; however, the improvement is greater in the physical training groups.
2. Conventional strength training has a greater positive effect on physical and psychological wellbeing than eccentric strength training.

Hypothesis 1: A repeated measures analysis with planned contrasts was chosen to test this hypothesis. Results yielded a significant main effect for session, $F(1, 35) = 15.694$, $p= .000$, indicating that all groups had experienced an increase in well-being over time (Figure 14). There was no significant main effect for training group ($F(2, 35) = .479$, $p= .623$) or interaction effect ($F(2, 35) = 1.883$, $p= .167$) (Table 23). In the planned contrasts, cognitive training was compared to physical training (both eccentric training and conventional strength training taken together as one group). This did not yield a significant result (Helmert contrast $p= .503$).

*Table 23: Repeated measures summary for overall well-being*

| Source | df | SS | MS | F | Sign. |
|---|---|---|---|---|---|
| Between subjects | | | | | |
| training group | 2 | 1348.947 | 674.473 | .479 | .623 |
| Error 1 | 35 | 49235.527 | 1406.729 | | |
| Within subjects | | | | | |
| Session | 1 | 5077.625 | 5077.625 | 15.694 | .000 |
| training group*session | 2 | 1218.571 | 609.286 | 1.883 | .167 |
| Error 2 | 35 | 11323.593 | 323.531 | | |

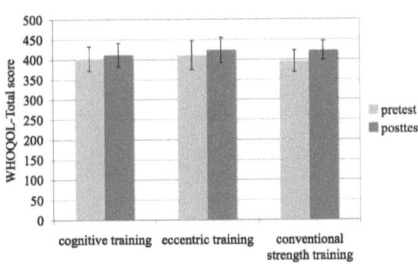

*Figure 14: Overall well-being in the three training groups prior and after the intervention*

Hypothesis 2: This hypothesis was tested with an independent samples t-test. The improvement in physical well-being in the eccentric group ($M_{ecc}$= 8.87, $SE_{ecc}$= 8.01) did not differ significantly from the improvement in the conventional muscle training group ($M_{con}$= 9.81, $SE_{con}$= 7.05, $t(23)$= -.31, $p$= .38 one-sided, $r$= .06). Neither did the improvement in the psychological wellbeing domain differ significantly between the two groups ($M_{ecc}$= 2.27, $SE_{ecc}$= 5.70, $M_{con}$= 3.57, $SE_{con}$= 5.39, $t(23)$= -.583, $p$= .28 one-sided, $r$= .12).

Therefore, it cannot be confirmed that conventional strength training has a greater positive effect on physical and psychological well-being than eccentric strength training.

**Hypothesis concerned with the interrelation of cognition and well-being**: An improvement in memory variables is predictive of an improvement in overall well-being.

The results of the regression analyses (Table 24) show that changes in the three memory tests Digit Span, Wechsler Memory Story and Free Recall explain 32.6% of variance in the change of well-being between test sessions. Only change in the Wechsler Memory Story turned out to be a significant predictor.

*Table 24: Regression summary for memory variables predicting change in psychological well-being*

| Variable | B | SEB | Beta | Sig. |
|---|---|---|---|---|
| Change in Digit Span total | 5.436 | 2.835 | .296 | .064 |
| Change in Wechsler Story | 1.987 | .952 | .295 | .044 |
| Change in Free Recall | -2.287 | 1.308 | -.271 | .089 |

Note: $R^2 = .33$, $N=37$

### 5.2.3 Summary of well-being results

Physical training, be it eccentric or conventional, is associated with an improvement in overall well-being. This improvement concerns physical as well as psychological well-being, with the increase being greater in the physical than in the psychological domain. Eccentric and conventional strength training did not differ with regard to their effect on physical and psychological well-being.

Cognitive training led to an increase in physical but not psychological well-being. There was no significant difference between physical and cognitive training in regard to improvement in overall well-being.

The changes from pre- to posttest in the memory measures Digit Span, Wechsler Story and Free Recall were found to explain 32% of variance in the pre-posttest change of overall well-being. The Wechsler Story as indicator of verbal episodic memory was the only significant predictor.

# 6 Discussion

In this thesis several research questions were pursued. The first question was whether eccentric exercise would have a positive effect on well-being and cognition. A second aim was to directly compare physical (i.e. eccentric and conventional strength training) and cognitive training in its effectiveness on well-being and cognition. Concerning the cognitive training, the focus lay on examining whether transfer effects could be achieved on non-trained cognitive tasks. Last but not least, exploratory analyses were conducted to find out which persons profited most from a given training.

As often in science, the results were not entirely clear-cut. In regard to the first question, whether eccentric exercise has a positive effect on well-being, there was a medium to large positive effect ($r=.50$) in overall well-being; however, this effect failed to reach statistical significance, probably due to the small sample size (n=11). There was, however, a significant increase in physical well-being at posttest. In view of this, one can assume that eccentric exercise does have a positive effect on well-being, at least on its physical components. This result fits well with the wealth of literature that has reported positive effects of different kinds of physical exercise on well-being (Arent et al., 2000; Netz et al., 2005; Norris et al., 1990). It has to be mentioned, however, that in our study, conventional strength training was even more successful in boosting well-being than eccentric strength training. There are several possible explanations for this finding: First of all, the conventional strength training was conducted in groups, whereas the participants of the eccentric training group were alone with a coach (who was a young person). It is possible that the social interaction and feeling of belonging to a group led to enhanced well-being in the conventional training group. A second reason could be that eccentric training appears less strenuous to the person working out than conventional training, due to the lower strain on the cardiovascular system. It is therefore possible that the mastery experience of the eccentric training group was smaller than the one of the conventional strength training group, leading to a smaller increase in well-being.

In addition to the question whether eccentric training would positively affect well-being, it was also of interest whether this type of training would have a positive effect on cognition. Due to the special characteristics of eccentric training, which demands that the participant constantly monitors his/her strength application on a computer screen and adjusts it accordingly, it was hypothesized that this training might have positive effects on executive functions, seeing as this constituted basically a dual task. However, the statistical analyses yielded no evidence for this hypothesis whatsoever. Eccentric training also did not lead to an improvement in memory; however, this had been expected. There was also only very scant evidence that eccentric training might lead to an improvement in speed. There was a medium to large effect in one speed measure (Reaction time), which failed to reach significance, probably due to the small sample size, but there was no effect in the second speed measure (Digit Symbol Task). The improvement in reaction time did not appear be due to a test-retest effect, as the performance of the other two training groups actually deteriorated. In view of these contradictory results, it is difficult to arrive at a definite conclusion whether eccentric training does lead to an improvement on speed measures or not. Clear is, however, that there seems to be no effect on executive functions. A possible explanation for this finding could be that a dual task combining strength regulation and attention (as the eccentric training can be perceived to be) is too different from a dual task containing perceptual identification and attention to yield transfer effects. Furthermore, one could even say that the eccentric training was not really a dual task, as the lines on the computer screen demanding attention were directly dependent on the strength application. In a more traditional understanding of dual tasks, the two tasks are usually completely unrelated.

A second main focus of this thesis was the direct comparison of physical and cognitive training in respect to their effects on well-being and cognition. So far, there is a distinct lack in literature about this topic. Our results show that the increase in overall well-being in the cognitive training group did not differ significantly from the increase in the physical training group. It was further hypothesized that physical training would mainly lead to an improvement in physical well-being, while cognitive training would lead to an improvement in psychological well-being. However, it turned out that both physical and cognitive training improved mainly physical well-being. Only the conventional strength training yielded an improvement in psychological well-being. Why did the cognitive training not improve psychological well-being? One possible answer is that the items of this scale of the WHOQOL-Bref assessed facets of psychological well-being that were not changed by a cognitive training. The psychological well-being domain consisted of six items. Two of these items were concerned with body image and sprituality, respectively, which both would not be expected to be changed by cognitive training (rather, body image might be changed by physical training). This left four items (positive feelings, negative feelings, self esteem, and concentration), only two of which were directly targeted by the cognitive training, namely self esteem (by stereotype activation) and concentration. A significant change in just these two items would probably not have been enough to create a statistical effect big enough to be detected with the present sample size.

With regard to comparing physical and cognitive training effects on cognition, cognitive training proved to be superior to physical training only with regard to improving Stroop performance. There was no difference with regard to other executive function measures. The Stroop task is considered to be a measure of inhibition. Therefore, it appears that cognitive training improved inhibitory function but not task coordination (as measured by dual task). At first sight, this may appear surprising. However, the working memory training was lacking certain characteristics that were inherent in the dual task of the testing situations. Even though the participants did have to remember a sequence of items (and had to continuously update this sequence) while making the upside down versus right side up decision, this task combination could partially be paced by the participants. Only once the participant had entered his decision about the orientation of one picture did the next picture appear. If the participant was too slow, he was reminded to work faster. However, there may still have been some leeway in the time allotted for deciding, allowing the participant to set his own pace. Therefore, while the timing of the two tasks constituting the dual task used during the pre- and posttest was completely independent of one another, this was not the case for the two tasks used in the cognitive training.

It is interesting to note that conventional strength training also led to an improvement in the Stroop task. Previous studies have yielded that aerobic training is beneficial for executive function (Kramer et al., 1999; Colcombe & Kramer, 2003). As was mentioned before, most trainings include a combination of anaerobic and aerobic exercise. The conventional strength training used in this study probably also had aerobic components (participants' heartrate was not monitored). If the aerobic characteristic was decisive for an improvement in executive function, this might explain why the conventional strength training group improved while the eccentric training group did not, seeing as the eccentric training was explicitly designed to put little strain on the cardiovascular system.

Concerning memory, the cognitive training was the only training to have a positive effect on memory function. A significant improvement in visual long-term memory was found. This could be due to the working memory training using visual material. It is surprising that there was no effect in the digit span measures, especially in digit span backwards. After all, digit span backwards, while differing from the working memory training in regard to material (verbal versus visual) and mode of presentation (auditive versus visual), has some commonalities with the working memory training. In both cases a sequence has to be remembered while the attention is directed at other information. It therefore appears that the differences between the two tasks weighed heavier than the commonalities.

Against expectation, there was also no effect of conventional strength training on memory (as opposed to Perrig-Chiello et al., 1998). However, there also other studies using conventional weight training that did not find any effects on memory (e.g. Moul, Goldman, & Warren, 1995). It is difficult to determine what is responsible for the different results, as the studies differ markedly in terms of duration of training, frequency of training and memory measures used for assessment.

The third main question of this thesis was whether the cognitive training would yield transfer effects. This question can be answer with a yes. There was a significant improvement from pretest to posttest in Stroop inhibition and Free Recall, even though these tasks were not trained. This improvement cannot be attributed to a simple retest-effect, as not all groups showed a significant increase in posttest scores. This result is remarkable considering the amount of cognitive training studies which failed to yield transfer effects. It is difficult to say what exactly is responsible for this effect. In view of the results of the working memory training by Klingberg and colleagues (2002), which yielded transfer effects, and the lack of transfer effects usually observed with other tpyes of training, it is likely that it is the working memory component of our cognitive training that is responsible for the observed transfer effects. This would be consistent with the view that working memory capacity is the basis for other memory functions, such as long term memory. More studies are needed to confirm these effects in other and especially bigger samples. However, for now it appears that working memory training is an excellent candidate for a memory training with older people that can yield transfer effects.

The results of this study showed that there was a lot of variation in the change from pretest to posttest. Some people profited immensely from the training, while others remained stable or even showed deterioration. In view of this, it was of interest to find out what prerequisites are necessary to profit from a training. Neither age, gender nor baseline intelligence were associated with subsequent improvement. However, a high baseline performance was associated with a tendency to decline, while a low baseline performance was associated with a tendency to improve at posttest (this held true for most memory measures, some of the executive function measures as well for all speed measures). This "regression to the mean" is a phenomenon that is quite often observed. This can be due to test characteristics, when tests are very lax in the low performance area and very stringent in the area of high performance, or when there are ceiling or floor effects at pretest However, we tried to avoid this problem by using raw scores only; furthermore, there were no ceiling or floor effects in the measures reported in this thesis. It therefore appears that in our case, the regression to the mean is due to sample characteristics rather than test characteristics.

Last but not least, what influence does the cognitive performance level have on well-being in the elderly? The regression analysis showed that changes in memory, especially in long-term episodic memory, are predictive of changes in well-being. This result lends credence to the complaints of older people, who often say that they are bothered by their memory problems. The results of this study show that an improvement in memory, such as can be achieved by a cognitive training, can also improve well-being in older people.

In sum, eccentric training has not been superior to conventional strength training with regard to improving well-being and cognition in the elderly. However, in view of the reduced cardiovascular strain that characterizes eccentric training, it may still be the most recommendable training for elderly with cardiovascular problems, possibly in combination with a cognitive training. Conventional strength training was effective in improving well-being as well as inhibitory function. The cognitive training used in the ExTrA study has yielded that it is possible to construct a training that is fun and interesting for the elderly and still produces a positive effect on non-trained memory tasks and inhibitory function. Furthermore, it has become clear that an improvement in memory function is predictive of an improvement in well-being.

*Limitations of the present study*
The greatest limitation of the present study was probably the small sample size (between 11 and 14 participants per group, total N=38). This sample size was determined by circumstantial constraints, such as the limited number of coaches available and that there was only one eccentric bike. Furthermore, the recruitment of healthy people over 80 who met our inclusion criteria and were willing to invest 90 minutes per week over a three month period proved much more difficult than first assumed. However, a bigger sample size would have made different analyses possible, such as factor analyses or structural equation modeling. Also, the statistical power would have been bigger, which would have allowed the detection of smaller effects. A second limitation of the study presented in this thesis is the bias in the sample. The participants were extremely fit and healthy for their age and cannot be considered representative for this age group as a whole. It is therefore difficult to say whether the results would also apply to a less "fit" sample. A third limitation is that this study has no real control group. All groups participated in some kind of training, there was no waiting-list group that was only

tested at pre- and posttest. This makes it impossible to estimate the effect of repeated testing[3]. Also, the group assignment was not completely random; for example, people who took blood thinning medication or had artificial joints (which were originally determined to lead to exclusion from the study) were assigned to the cognitive training group, as there were not enough participants. Another limitation concerned the cognitive training. It was a multi-component training, which is more interesting for participants and therefore most likely improves compliance. However, with such a training it is impossible to say which component was responsible for the observed effects. More studies which examine the different components singly would be needed to answer this question. It is also possible that a different well-being measure might have yielded better results. Perrig-Chiello (1997) or Ryff (1989) both created well-being measures that included mastery. It would have been interesting to see if one or several of the training interventions increased participants' sense of mastery.

*Future research questions*

For future research it would be interesting to see whether a combination of physical and cognitive training would potentiate the effects. It is also of interest whether certain effects observed in the eccentric training group would reach statistical significance with a bigger sample size. To this purpose, more people were recruited, trained and tested in an extension of the original study. The results of this as well as the results of a no-training control group, which was also assessed post hoc, are still pending. One other question concerns the duration of the observed effects. Would the improvement still hold after a year? Even though there was a follow-up testing in the ExTrA study after a year, it is difficult to arrive at a conclusion, due to the amount of intervening variables. Some people continued to exercise after the official training had ended, others did not. Some lost partners, some were hospitalized or severly ill, some moved into assisted living. Furthermore, the medications had changed with quite a few of the participants. With the present small sample size it was impossible to control for all of these variables, and it was therefore decided not to report the results of the follow-up examination. However, for future studies with bigger samples it would be of great interest to see if there are lasting effects of physical and cognitive training. Last but not least, the ExtrA project is extraordinary in respect that it would allow to put cognitive and physical changes in old age into context. The results from blood screenings, electrocardiograms, muscle biopsies etc. may yield further insights concerning why certain people experience a deterioration of cognitive functioning in old age while others do not.

---

[3] a control group which only underwent pre- and posttest testing has been assessed post hoc; furthermore, more people underwent the eccentric training intervention to increase the sample size. However, these results will not be included in this study due to time constraints.

The results from this thesis have once again shown very clearly that there is a great interindividual variance in aging and age-associated decline. Old age is not period of life when everything stagnates - rather, there is an immense potential for development. Even though plasticity may be reduced in comparison to younger people, it is nevertheless still present in the elderly, and offers a tremendous opportunity. I'd like to close with a quote which puts this into words better than I ever could:

*"For age is opportunity no less*
*Than youth itself, though in another dress,*
*And as the evening twilight fades away,*
*The sky is filled with stars invisible by day."*
—Henry Wadsworth Longfellow

# References

Abeles, R. P., Gift, H. C., & Ory, M. G. (Eds.). (1994). *Aging and quality of life*. New York: Springer.

Anderson, B., & Rutledge, V. (1996). Age and hemisphere effects on dendritic structure. *Brain, 119 ( Pt 6)*, 1983-1990.

Angermeyer, M. C., Kilian, R., & Matschinger, H. (2000). *WHOQOL-100 und WHOQOL-BREF: Handbuch der deutschsprachigen Version der WHO Instrumente zur Erfassung von Lebensqualität*. Göttingen: Hogrefe.

Arent, S. M., Landers, D. M., & Etnier, J. L. (2000). The effects of exercise on mood in older adults: A meta-analytic review. *Journal of Aging and Physical Activity, 8*, 407-430.

Argyle, M. (1999). Causes and correlates of happiness. In D. Kahneman, E. Diener & N. Schwarz (Eds.), *Well-being: The foundations of hedonic psychology* (pp. 353-373). New York: Russell Sage.

Atkinson, R. C., & Shiffrin, R. M. (1968). Human memory: A proposed system and its control processes. In K. W. Spence (Ed.), *The psychology of learning and motivation: Advances in research and theory* (pp. 89-195). New York: Academic Press.

Babyak, M. A., Blumenthal, J. A., Herman, S., Khatri, P., Doraiswamy, M., Moore, K. A., et al. (2000). Exercise treatment for major depression: Maintenance of therapeutic benefit at 10 months. *Psychosomatic Medicine, 62*(5), 633-638.

Baddeley, A. (2000). The episodic buffer: a new component of working memory? *Trends in Cognitive Sciences, 4*(11), 417-423.

Baddeley, A., & Hitch, G. J. (1974). Working memory. In G. A. Bower (Ed.), *The psychology of learning and motivation: advances in research and theory* (Vol. 8, pp. 47-89). New York: Psychology Press.

Baeumler, G. (1985). *Farbe-Wort-Interferenztest (FWIT)*. Göttingen: Hogrefe.

Ball, K., Berch, D. B., Helmers, K. F., Jobe, J. B., Leveck, M. D., Marsiske, M., et al. (2002). Effects of cognitive training interventions with older adults. *Journal of the American Medical Association, 288*(18), 2271-2281.

Baltes, M., Maas, I., Wims, H.-U., & Borchelt, M. (1996). Alltagskompetenz im Alter: Theoretische Überlegungen und empirische Befunde. In K. U. Mayer & P. B. Baltes (Eds.), *Die Berliner Altersstudie* (pp. 525-542). Berlin: Akademie-Verlag.

Baltes, P. B., & Baltes, M. (1990). Psychological perspectives on successful aging: The model of selective optimization with compensation. In P. B. Baltes & M. M. Baltes (Eds.), *Successful aging* (pp. 1-27). Cambridge: Cambridge University Press.

Barchas, J. D., & Freedman, D. X. (1963). Brain amines: Response to physiological stress. *Biochemistry and Pharmacology, 12*, 1232-1235.

Bargh, J. A., Chen, M., & Burrows, L. (1996). Automaticity of social behavior: direct effects of trait construct and stereotype-activation on action. *Journal of Personality and Social Psychology, 71*(2), 230-244.

Beason-Held, L. L., & Horwitz, B. (2002). Aging Brain. In V. S. Ramachandran (Ed.), *Encyclopedia of the Human Brain* (Vol. 1, pp. 43-57). San Diego, CA: Academic Press.

Bee, H. L., & Bjorklund, B. R. (2004). *The journey of adulthood* (5 ed.). Upper Saddle River, NJ: Pearson/Prentice Hall.

Black, J. E., Isaacs, K. R., Anderson, B. J., Alcantara, A. A., & Greenough, W. T. (1990). Learning causes synaptogenesis, whereas motor activity causes angiogenesis, in cerebellar cortex of adult rats. *Proceedings of the National Academy of Sciences, 87*, 5568-5572.

Blane, D., Higgs, P., Hyde, M., & Wiggins, R. D. (2004). Life course influences on quality of life in early old age. *Social Science and Medicine, 58*, 2171-2179.

Blumenthal, J. A., Babyak, M. A., Moore, K. A., Craighead, W. E., Herman, S., Khatri, P., et al. (1999). Effects of exercise training on older patients with major depression. *Archives of Internal Medicine, 159*, 2349-2356.

Blumenthal, J. A., Emery, C. F., Madden, D. J., Schniebolk, S., Walsh-Riddle, M., George, L. K., et al. (1991). Long-term effects of exercise on psychological functioning in older men and women. *Journal of Gerontology: Psychological Sciences, 46*(6), 352-361.

Boone, K. B., Miller, B. L., Lesser, I. M., Mehringer, C. M., Hill-Gutierrez, E., Goldberg, M. A., et al. (1992). Neuropsychological correlates of white-matter lesions in healthy elderly subjects. A threshold effect. *Archives of Neurology, 49*(5), 549-554.

Bortz, W. M., Angwin, P., Mefford, I. N., Boarder, M. R., Noyce, N., & Barchas, J. D. (1981). Catecholamines, dopamine, and endorphin levels during extreme exercise. *New England Journal of Medicine, 305*, 466-467.

Bradburn, N. M., & Caplovitz, D. (1965). *Reports of happiness*. Chicago: Aldine.

Brandtstädter, J. (2002). Searching for paths to successful development and aging: integrating developmental and action-theoretical perspectives. In L. Pulkkinen & A. Caspi (Eds.), *Paths to successful development. Personality in the life course* (pp. 380-408). Cambridge: Cambridge University Press.

Brickman, P., & Campbell, D. T. (1971). Hedonic relativism and planning the good society. In M. H. Appley (Ed.), *Adaptation level theory: A symposium* (pp. 287-302). New York: Academic Press.

Brown, L. A., Shumway-Cook, A., & Woollacott, M. H. (1999). Attentional demands and postural recovery: the effects of aging. *Journal of Gerontology: Biological Sciences, 54*, 165-171.

Buchner, A., Faul, F., & Erdfelder, E. (1997). G*Power: A priori, post hoc, analyses for the Macintosh (Version 2.1.2). Trier, Germany: University of Trier.

Burgess, P. W. (1997). Theory and methodology in executive function research. In P. Rabbitt (Ed.), *Methodology of frontal and executive function* (pp. 81-116). Hove, U.K.: Psychology Press.

Buschkuehl, M. (2007). Arbeitsgedächtnistraining [working memory training]. Unpublished doctoral dissertation. University of Bern, Switzerland.

Caprio-Prevette, M. D., & Fry, P. S. (1996). Memory enhancement program for community-based older adults: development and evaluation. *Experimental Aging Research, 22*(3), 281-303.

Cerella, J. (1985). Information processing rates in the elderly. *Psychological Bulletin, 98*, 67-83.

Cerella, J. (1990). Aging and information processing rate. In J. E. Birren & K. W. Schaie (Eds.), *Handbook of psychology of aging* (3 ed., pp. 201-222). New York: Academic Press.

Colcombe, S., Erickson, K. I., Raz, N., Webb, A., Cohen, N. J., McAuley, E., et al. (2003). Aerobic fitness reduces brain tissue loss in aging humans. *Journal of Gerontology: Medical Sciences, 58A*(2), 176-180.

Colcombe, S., & Kramer, A. F. (2003). Fitness effects on the cognitive function of older adults: a meta-analytic study. *Psychological Science, 14*(2), 125-130.

Courchesne, E., Chisum, H. J., Townsend, J., Cowles, A., Covington, J., Egaas, B., et al. (2000). Normal brain development and aging: quantitative analysis at in vivo MR imaging in healthy volunteers. *Radiology, 216*(3), 672-682.

Cowan, N. (2005). *Working memory capacity*. New York: Psychology Press.

Craft, L. L. (2005). Exercise and clinical depression: examining two psychological mechanisms. *Psychology of Sport and Exercise, 6*, 151-171.

Craik, F. I., & Byrd, M. (1982). Aging and cognitive deficits: The role of attentional resources. In F. I. Craik & S. E. Trehub (Eds.), *Aging and cognitive processes* (pp. 191-211). New York: Plenum Press.

Dani, S. U., Pittella, J. E., Boehme, A., Hori, A., & Schneider, B. (1997). Progressive formation of neuritic plaques and neurofibrillary tangles is exponentially related to age and neuronal size. A morphometric study of three geographically distinct series of aging people. *Dementia and Geriatric Cognitive Disorders, 8*(4), 217-227.

Davey, C. P. (1973). Physical exertion and mental performance. *Ergonomics, 16*, 595-599.

Davis, H. P., & Bernstein, P. A. (1992). Age-related changes in explicit and implicit memory. In L. R. Squire & N. Butters (Eds.), *Neuropsychology of memory*. Hillsdale: Guilford Press.

de Groot, J. C., de Leeuw, F. E., Oudkerk, M., van Gijn, J., Hofman, A., Jolles, J., et al. (2000). Cerebral white matter lesions and cognitive function: the Rotterdam Scan Study. *Annals of Neurology, 47*(2), 145-151.

Diener, E. (1984). Subjective well-being. *Psychological Bulletin, 95*, 542-575.

Diener, E., & Fujita, F. (1995). Resources, personal strivings, and subjective well-being: A nomothetic and idiographic approach. *Journal of Personality and Social Psychology, 68*(5), 926-935.

Diener, E., & Lucas, R. E. (1999). Personality and subjective well-being. In D. Kahneman, E. Diener & N. Schwarz (Eds.), *Well-being: The foundations of hedonic psychology* (pp. 213-229). New York: Russell Sage.

Diener, E., Lucas, R. E., & Scollon, C. N. (2006). Beyond the hedonic treadmill: Revising the adaptation theory of well-being. *American Psychologist, 61*(4), 305-314.

Diener, E., Sandvik, E., & Larsen, R. J. (1985). Age and sex effects for affect intensity. *Developmental Psychology, 21*, 542-546.

Diener, E., & Suh, E. M. (1998). Subjective well-being and age: An international analysis. In K. W. Schaie & M. P. Lawton (Eds.), *Annual Review of Gerontology and Geriatrics* (Vol. 17, pp. 304-324). New York: Springer.

Diener, E., Suh, E. M., Lucas, R. E., & Smith, H. L. (1999). Subjective well-being: Three decades of progress. *Psychological Bulletin, 125*(2), 276-302.

Drevets, W. C., & Raichle, M. E. (1992). Neuroanatomical circuits in depression: Implications for treatment mechanisms. *Psychopharmalogical Bulletin, 28*, 261-273.

Dustman, R. E., Ruhling, R. O., Russell, E. M., Shearer, D. E., Bonekat, H. W., Shigeoka, J. W., et al. (1984). Aerobic exercise training and improved neuropsychological function of older individuals. *Neurobiology of Aging, 5*, 35-42.

Emery, C. F., & Gatz, M. (1990). Psychological and cognitive effects of an exercise program for community-residing older adults. *The Gerontologist, 30*(2), 184-188.

Ericsson, K. A., & Kintsch, W. (1995). Long-term working memory. *Psychological Review, 102*, 211-245.

Erikson, E. H. (1982). *The Life Cycle Completed: A Review*. New York: Norton.

Etnier, J. L., Salazar, W., Landers, D. M., Petruzzello, S. J., Han, M., & Nowell, P. (1997). The influence of physical fitness and exercise upon cognitive functioning: A meta-analysis. *Journal of Sport & Exercise Psychology, 19*, 249-277.

Fabre, C., Chamari, K., Mucci, P., Masse-Biron, J., & Prefaut, C. (2002). Improvement of cognitive function by mental and/or individualized aerobic training in healthy elderly subjects. *International Journal of Sports Medicine, 23*(6), 415-421.

Fabre, C., Masse-Biron, J., Chamari, K., Varray, A., Mucci, P., & Prefaut, C. (1999). Evaluation of quality of life in elderly healthy subjects after aerobic and/or mental training. *Archives of Gerontology and Geriatrics, 28*, 9-22.

Field, A. (2005). *Discovering statistics using SPSS* (2 ed.). London: Sage.

Fischer, B., Lehrl, S., & Grässel, E. (2002). *Gehirn-Jogging: Übungsprogramm Band 4*. Ebersberg: Vless.

Fischer, B., Lehrl, S., & Kindl, I. (1998). *Gehirn-Jogging: Übungsaufgaben Band 5*. Ebersberg: Vless.

Fischer, B., Lehrl, S., & Wurzer, I. (1992). *Gehirn-Jogging: Übungsprogramm 1*. Ebersberg: Vless.

Fischer, B., Lehrl, S., & Wurzer, I. (1993). *Gehirn-Jogging: Übungsprogramm Band 2*. Ebersberg: Vless.

Fischer, B., Lehrl, S., & Wurzer, I. (1997). *Gehirn-Jogging: Übungsprogramm Band 3*. Ebersberg: Vless.

Fleischmann, U. M., & Oswald, W. D. (1997-1999). *Nürnberger-Alters-Inventar (NAI)* (4 ed.). Göttingen: Hogrefe.

Floyd, M., & Scogin, F. (1997). Effects of memory training on the subjective memory functioning and mental health of older adults: A meta-analysis. *Psychology and Aging, 12*(1), 150-161.

Flynn, R. (1972). Numerical performance as a function of prior exercise and aerobic capacity for elementary school boys. *Research Quarterly, 43*, 16-22.

Fortin, M., Bravo, G., Hudon, C., Vanasse, A., & Lapointe, L. (2005). Prevalence of multimorbidity among adults seen in family practice. *Annals of Family Medicine, 3*(3), 223-228.

Fozard, J. L., & Gordon-Salant, S. (2001). Sensory and perceptual changes with aging. In J. E. Birren & K. W. Schaie (Eds.), *Handbook of the Psychology of Aging* (5 ed., pp. 241-266). San Diego: Academic Press.

Frederick, S., & Loewenstein, G. (1999). Hedonic Adaptation. In D. Kahneman, E. Diener & N. Schwarz (Eds.), *Well-being: The foundations of a hedonic psychology* (pp. 302-329). New York: Russell Sage.

Fries, J. F. (2005). The compression of morbidity. *The Milbank Quarterly, 83*(4), 801-823.

Gatz, M., & Karel, M. J. (1993). Individual Change in Perceived Control over 20 Years. *International Journal of Behavioral Development, 16*(2), 305-322.

Gill, T. M., Baker, T. I., Gottschalk, M., Peduzzi, P. N., Allore, H., & Byers, A. (2002). A program to prevent functional decline in physically frail, elderly persons who live at home. *New England Journal of Medicine, 347*, 1068-1074.

Gill, T. M., Baker, T. I., Gottschalk, M., Peduzzi, P. N., Allore, H., & Van Ness, P. H. (2004). A rehabilitation program for the prevention of functional decline: Effect of higher-level physical function. *Archives of Physical Medicine and Rehabilitation, 85*, 1043-1049.

Grundy, E., & Bowling, A. (1999). Enhancing the quality of extended life years. Identification of the oldest old with a very good and very poor quality of life. *Aging and Mental Health, 3*, 199-212.

Gupta, V. P., Sharma, T. R., & Jaspal, S. S. (1974). Physical activity and efficiency of mental work. *Perceptual and Motor Skills, 38*, 205-206.

Gutin, B., & DiGennaro, J. (1968a). Effect of a treadmill run to exhaustion on performance of simple addition. *Research Quarterly, 39*, 958-964.

Gutin, B., & DiGennaro, J. (1968b). Effect of one-minute and five-minute step-ups on performance of simple addition. *Research Quarterly, 39*, 81-85.

Härting, C., Markowitsch, H. J., Neufeld, H., Calabrese, P., Deisinger, K., & Kessler, J. (Eds.). (2000). *WMS-R: Wechsler Gedächtnistest*. Bern: Huber.

Hasher, L., & Zacks, R. T. (1988). Working memory, comprehension, and aging: A review and a new view. In G. A. Bower (Ed.), *The Psychology of Learning and Motivation* (Vol. 22, pp. 193-225). New York: Academic Press.

Hasher, L., Zacks, R. T., & Rahhal, T. A. (1999). Timing, instructions, and inhibitory control: Some missing factors in the age and memory debate. *Gerontology, 45*, 355-357.

Hassmen, P., Ceci, R., & Backman, L. (1992). Exercise for older women: a training method and its influences on physical and cognitive performance. *European Journal of Applied Physiology, 64*, 460-466.

Hausdorff, J. M., Levy, B. R., & Wei, J. Y. (1999). The power of ageism on physical function of older persons: reversibility of age-related gait changes. *Journal of the American Geriatrics Society, 47*(11), 1346-1349.

Hawkins, H. L., Kramer, A. F., & Capaldi, D. (1992). Aging, exercise, and attention. *Psychology and Aging, 7*(4), 643-653.

Heady, B., Veenhoven, R., & Wearing, A. (1991). Top-down versus bottom-up theories of subjective well-being. *Social Indicators Research, 24*, 81-100.

Hellström, G., Fischer-Colbrie, W., Wahlgren, N. G., & Jogestrand, T. (1996). Carotid artery blood flow and middle cerebral artery blood flow velocity during physical exercise. *Journal of Applied Physiology, 81*(1), 413-418.

Helmchen, H., Baltes, M., Geiselmann, B., Kanowski, S., Linden, M., Reischies, F. M., et al. (1996). Psychische Erkrankungen im Alter. In K. U. Mayer & P. B. Baltes (Eds.), *Die Berliner Altersstudie*. Berlin: Akademie Verlag.

Hess, T. M., Hinson, J. T., & Statham, J. A. (2004). Explicit and implicit stereotype activation effects on memory: do age and awareness moderate the impact of priming? *Psychology and Aging, 19*(3), 495-505.

Hill, R. D., Storandt, M., & Malley, M. (1993). The impact of long-term exercise training on psychological function in older adults. *Journal of Gerontology: Psychological Sciences, 48*(1), 12-17.

Hill, R. D., Storandt, M., & Simeone, C. (1990). The effects of memory skills training and incentives on free recall in older learners. *Journal of Gerontology, 45*(6), P227-232.

Holahan, C. K., Holahan, C. J., & Wonacott, N. L. (2001). Psychological well-being at age 80: Health-related and psychosocial factors. *Journal of Mental Health and Aging, 7*(4), 395-411.

Hortobagyi, T., Money, J., Zheng, D., Dudek, R., Fraser, D., & Dohm, L. (2002). Muscle Adaptations to 7 Days of Exercise in Young and Older Humans: Eccentric Overload Versus Standard Resistive Training. *Journal of Aging and Physical Activity, 10*(3), 290-305.

Ide, K., & Secher, N. H. (2000). Cerebral blood flow and metabolism during exercise. *Progress in Neurobiology, 61*, 397-414.

Jahn, T. (2004). Neuropsychologie der Demenz. In S. Lautenbacher & S. Gauggel (Eds.), *Neuropsychologie psychischer Störungen* (pp. 301-338). Berlin: Springer.

Jones, T. G., Rapport, L. J., Hanks, R. A., Lichtenberg, P. A., & Telmet, K. (2003). Cognitive and psychosocial predictors of subjective well-being in urban older adults. *The Clinical Neuropsychologist, 17*(1), 3-18.

Jopp, D., & Smith, J. (2006). Resources and life-management strategies as determinants of successful aging: on the protective effect of selection, optimization and compensation. *Psychology and Aging, 21*(2), 253-265.

Kahn, R. L., & Juster, F. T. (2002). Well-being: concepts and measures. *Journal of Social Issues, 58*(4), 627-644.

Kessler, J., & Kalbe, E. (2000). Gerontoneuropsychologie - Grundlagen und Pathologie. In W. Sturm, M. Herrmann & C.-W. Wallesch (Eds.), *Lehrbuch der klinischen Neuropsychologie* (pp. 648-662). Lisse, NL: Swets & Zeitlinger.

Kester, J. D., Benjamin, A. S., Castel, A. D., & Craik, F. I. (2002). Memory in elderly people. In A. Baddeley, M. D. Kopelman & B. A. Wilson (Eds.), *The handbook of memory disorders*. London: John Wiley & Sons.

Ketcham, C. J., & Stelmach, G. E. (2001). Age-related declines in motor control. In J. E. Birren & K. W. Schaie (Eds.), *Handbook of the psychology of aging* (5 ed., pp. 313-348). San Diego: Academic Press.

King, A. C., Taylor, C. B., & Haskell, W. L. (1993). Effects of differing intensities and formats of 12 months of exercise training on psychological outcomes in older adults. *Health Psychology, 12*(4), 292-300.

Klauer, K. J. (2002). *Denksport für Ältere: Geistig fit bleiben*. Bern: Hans Huber.

Kliegl, R., & Baltes, P. B. (1991). Testing-the-limits kognitiver Entwicklungskapazität in einer Gedächtnisleistung. *Zeitschrift für Psychologie, Supplement 11*, 84-92.

Kliegl, R., Smith, J., & Baltes, P. B. (1989). Testing-the-limits and the study of adult age differences in cognitive plasticity of a mnemonic skill. *Developmental Psychology, 25*, 247-256.

Kling, V. (1996). Kognitive Leistungsmessung bei älteren Menschen. Unveröffentlichte Dissertation: Universität Bern, Schweiz.

Klingberg, T., Forssberg, H., & Westerberg, H. (2002). Training of working memory in children with ADHD. *Journal of Clinical and Experimental Neuropsychology, 24*(6), 781-791.

Knopf, M. (2001). Optimierung des Gedächtnisses älterer Menschen durch Training. In K. J. Klauer (Ed.), *Handbuch kognitives Training* (pp. 491-512). Göttingen: Hogrefe.

Kozma, A., Stones, M. J., & McNeil, J. K. (1991). *Psychological well-being in later life*. Toronto: Butterworths.

Kramer, A. F., Hahn, S., Cohen, N. J., Banich, M. T., McAuley, E., Harrison, C. R., et al. (1999). Ageing, fitness and neurocognitive function. *Nature, 400*(6743), 418-419.

Kunzmann, U., Little, T., & Smith, J. (2000). Is age-related stability of subjective well-being a paradox? Cross-sectional findings from the Berlin Aging Study. *Psychology and Aging, 15*(3), 511-526.

Lachman, M. E. (1991). Perceived control over memory aging: Developmental and intervention perspectives. *Journal of Social Issues, 47*(4), 159-175.

Lawlor, D. A., & Hopker, S. W. (2001). The effectiveness of exercise as an intervention in the management of depression: systematic review and meta-regression analysis of randomized controlled trials. *British Medical Journal, 322*, 763-767.

Lehr, U. (2003). *Psychologie des Alterns* (10 ed.). Wiebelsheim: Quelle & Meyer.

Lehrl, S. (1989). *Mehrfachwahl-Wortschatz-Intelligenztest*. Erlangen: Perimed.

Lehrl, S., Merz, J., Burkhard, G., & Fischer, S. (1991). *Mehrfachwahl-Wortschatz-Intelligenztest (MWT-A)*. Erlangen: Perimed.

Leppert, K., Gunzelmann, T., Schumacher, J., Strauss, B., & Brähler, E. (2005). Resilienz als protektives Persönlichkeitsmerkmal im Alter. *Psychotherapie, Psychosomatik, Medizinische Psychologie, 55*, 365-369.

Levy, B. (1996). Improving memory in old age through implicit self-stereotyping. *Journal of Personality and Social Psychology, 71*(6), 1092-1107.

Lezak, M. D. (1995). *Neuropsychological Assessment* (3rd ed.). New York: Oxford University Press.

Madden, D. J., Blumenthal, J. A., Allen, P. A., & Emery, C. F. (1989). Improving aerobic capacity in healthy older adults does not necessarily lead to improved cogntive performance. *Psychology and Aging, 4*(3), 307-320.

Maddox, G. L. (1963). Activity and morale: A longitudinal study of selected elderly subjects. *Social Forces, 42*, 195-204.

Martin, M., & Kliegel, M. (2005). *Psychologische Grundlagen der Gerontologie* (Vol. Band 3). Stuttgart: Kohlhammer.

Masliah, E., Mallory, M., Hansen, L., DeTeresa, R., & Terry, R. D. (1993). Quantitative synaptic alterations in the human neocortex during normal aging. *Neurology, 43*(1), 192-197.

McAuley, E., Blissmer, B., Marquez, D. X., Jerome, G. J., Kramer, A. F., & Katula, J. (2000). Social relations, physical activity, and well-being in older adults. *Preventive Medicine, 31*, 608-617.

McAuley, E., & Rudolph, D. (1995). Physical activity, aging, and psychological well-being. *Journal of Aging and Physical Activity, 3*, 67-96.

McNeil, J. K., LeBlanc, E. M., & Joyner, M. (1991). The effect of exercise on depressive symptoms in the moderately depressed elderly. *Psychology and Aging, 6*(3), 487-488.

Meier, B. (1999). Altersbedingte Veränderungen in der Verarbeitungskapazität. In P. Perrig-Chiello, H. B. Staehelin & W. J. Perrig (Eds.), *Wohlbefinden, Gesundheit und kognitive Kompetenz im Alter* (pp. 123-130). Bern: Haupt.

Meier, B., & Perrig, W. J. (2000). Low reliability of perceptual priming: Consequences for the interpretation of functional dissociations between explicit and implicit memory. *The Quarterly Journal of Experimental Psychology, 53A*(1), 211-233.

Mitchell, J. B., Flynn, M. G., Goldfarb, A. H., Ben-Ezra, V., & Copman, T. L. (1990). The effect of training on the norepinephrine response at rest and during exercise in 5° and 20°C environments *The Journal of Sports Medicine and Physical Fitness, 30*, 235-240.

Moeller, J. R., Ishikawa, T., Dhawan, V., Spetsieris, P., Mandel, F., Alexander, G. E., et al. (1996). The metabolic topography of normal aging. *Journal of Cerebral Blood Flow and Metabolism, 16*(3), 385-398.

Mohs, R. C., Ashman, T. A., Jantzen, K., Albert, M., Brandt, J., Gordon, B., et al. (1998). A study of the efficacy of a comprehensive memory enhancement program in healthy elderly persons. *Psychiatry Research, 77*(3), 183-195.

Molinari, V., & Niederehe, G. (1984-85). Locus of control, depression, and anxiety in young and old adults: a comparison study. *International Journal of Aging and Human Development, 20*(1), 41-52.

Moul, J. L., Goldman, B., & Warren, B. (1995). Physical activity and cognitive performance in the older population. *Journal of Aging and Physical Activity, 3*, 135-145.

Mueller, E. A., Moore, M. M., Kerr, D. C., Sexton, G., Camicioli, R. M., Howieson, D. B., et al. (1998). Brain volume preserved in healthy elderly through the eleventh decade. *Neurology, 51*(6), 1555-1562.

Naveh-Benjamin, M., Guez, J., Kilb, A., & Reedy, S. (2004). The associative memory deficit of older adults: Further support using face-name associations. *Psychology and Aging, 19*(3), 541-546.

Neely Stigsdotter, A., & Bäckman, L. (1993). Long-term maintenance of gains from memory training in older adults: Two 3 1/2-year follow-up studies. *Journal of Gerontology: Psychological Sciences, 48*(5), P233-P237.

Neeper, S. A., Gomez-Pinilla, F., Choi, J., & Cotman, C. W. (1995). Exercise and brain neurotrophins. *Nature, 373*, 109.

Netz, Y., Wu, M.-J., Becker, B. J., & Tenenbaum, G. (2005). Physical activity and psychological well-being in advanced age: A meta-analysis of intervention studies. *Psychology and Aging, 20*(2), 272-284.

Newman, B., & Newman, P. (1995). *Development through life: A psychosocial approach* (6 ed.). Brooks/Cole: Pacific Grove, CA.

Noice, H., Noice, T., Perrig-Chiello, P., & Perrig, W. (1999). Improving memory in older adults by instructiong them in professional actors' learning strategies. *Applied Cognitive Psychology, 13*(4), 315-328.

Nolen-Hoeksema, S. (1991). Responses to depression and their effects on the duration of depressive episodes. *Journal of Abnormal Psychology, 100*(4), 569-582.

Norris, R., Carroll, D., & Cochrane, R. (1990). The effects of aerobic training and anaerobic training on fitness, blood pressure, and psychological stress and well-being. *Journal of Psychosomatic Research, 34*(4), 367-375.

North, T. C., McCullagh, P., & Tran, Z. V. (1990). Effects of exercise on depression. *Exercise and Sport Science Reviews, 18*, 379-415.

Okumiya, K., Matsubayashi, K., Wada, T., Kimura, S., Doi, Y., & Ozawa, T. (1996). Effects of exercise on neurobehavioral function in community-dwelling older people more than 75 years of age. *Journal of the American Geriatrics Society, 44*(5), 569-572.

Oswald, W. D. (Ed.). (1998). *Gedächtnistraining: ein Programm für Seniorengruppen.* Göttingen: Hogrefe.

Oswald, W. D., Rupprecht, R., Gunzelmann, T., & Tritt, K. (1996). The SIMA-project: Effects of 1 year cognitive and psychomotor training on cognitive abilities of the elderly. *Behavioural Brain Research, 78*, 67-72.

Pantoni, L., & Garcia, J. H. (1995). The significance of cerebral white matter abnormalities 100 years after Binswanger's report. A review. *Stroke, 26*(7), 1293-1301.

Perri, S. I., & Templer, D. I. (1985). The effects of an aerobic exercise program on psychological variables in older adults. *International Journal of Aging and Human Development, 20*(3), 167-172.

Perrig, W. J., Kling, V., Meier, B., Hofer, D., Perrig-Chiello, P., Ruch, M., et al. (1994). *Computerunterstützter Gedächtnis-Funktions-Test (C-GFT).* Basel: Universität Basel.

Perrig, W. J., Meier, B., & Ruch-Monachon, M. (1999). Veränderungen der impliziten und expliziten Gedächtnisfunktionen im Alter. In P. Perrig-Chiello, H. B. Staehelin & W. J. Perrig (Eds.), *Wohlbefinden, Gesundheit und kognitive Kompetenz im Alter* (pp. 119-123). Bern: Haupt.

Perrig, W. J., & Perrig, P. (1993). Life-span aspects in explicit and implicit memory. *The German Journal of Psychology, 17*, 307-309.

Perrig, W. J., & Perrig-Chiello, P. (1993). Implizites Gedächtnis: unwillkürlich, entwicklungsresistent und altersunabhängig? *Zeitschrift für Entwicklungspsychologie und Pädagogische Psychologie, XXV*(1), 29-47.

Perrig, W. J., & Perrig-Chiello, P. (1999). Zusammenhang zwischen subjektiver und objektiver Gesundheit und Wohlbefinden und Autonomie - oder: Die Regulation des Wohlbefindens. In P. Perrig-Chiello, H. B. Staehelin & W. J. Perrig (Eds.), *Wohlbefinden, Gesundheit und kognitive Kompetenz im Alter* (pp. 78-82). Bern: Haupt.

Perrig-Chiello, P. (1997). *Wohlbefinden im Alter. Körperliche, psychische und soziale Determinanten und Ressourcen.* München: Juventa Verlag.

Perrig-Chiello, P. (1999). Subjektive Gesundheit und Kotrollüberzeugungen. In P. Perrig-Chiello, H. B. Staehelin & W. J. Perrig (Eds.), *Wohlbefinden, Gesundheit und kognitive Kompetenz im Alter* (pp. 27-33). Bern: Haupt.

Perrig-Chiello, P. (2000). Control beliefs, health, and well-being in elderly. In W. Perrig & A. Grob (Eds.), *Control of human behavior, mental processes, and consciousness: Essays in honor of the 60th birthday of August Flammer.* Mahwah, NJ: Lawrence Erlbaum Associates.

Perrig-Chiello, P., Perrig, W. J., Ehrsam, R., Staehelin, H. B., & Krings, F. (1998). The effects of resistance training on well-being and memory in elderly volunteers. *Age and Ageing, 27*, 469-475.

Perrig-Chiello, P., Perrig, W. J., & Staehelin, H. B. (1999). Health control beliefs in old age-relationship with subjective and objective health and health behavior. *Psychology, Health, and Medicine, 4*, 83-95.

Perrig-Chiello, P., Perrig, W. J., Uebelbacher, A., & Staehelin, H. B. (2006). Impact of physical and psychological resources on functional autonomy in old age. *Psychology, Health & Medicine, 11*(4), 470-482.

Perrig-Chiello, P., Staehelin, H. B., & Ehrsam, R. (1999). Gesundheitsverhalten. In P. Perrig-Chiello, H. B. Staehelin & W. J. Perrig (Eds.), *Wohlbefinden, Gesundheit und kognitive Kompetenz im Alter* (pp. 83-92). Bern: Haupt.

Perrig-Chiello, P., Staehelin, H. B., & Perrig, W. J. (Eds.). (1999). *Wohlbefinden, Gesundheit und kognitive Kompetenz im Alter.* Bern: Haupt.

Phillips, W. T., M., K., & King, A. C. (2003). Physical activity as a nonpharmalogical treatment for depression: A review. *Complementary health practice review, 8*(2), 139-152.

Price, J. L., & Morris, J. C. (1999). Tangles and plaques in nondemented aging and "preclinical" Alzheimer's disease. *Annals of Neurology, 45*(3), 358-368.

Puts, M. T. E., Lips, P., Ribbe, M. W., & Deeg, D. J. H. (2005). The effect of frailty on residential/nursing home admission in the Netherlands independent of chronic diseases and functional limitations. *European Journal of Ageing, 2*, 264-274.

Rahhal, T. A., Colcombe, S. J., & Hasher, L. (2001). Instructional manipulations and age differences in memory: now you see them, now you don't. *Psychology and Aging, 16*(4), 697-706.

Ransford, C. (1982). A role for amines in the antidepressant effect of exercise: a review. *Medical Science in Sports, 14*, 1-10.

Resnick, S. M., Pham, D. L., Kraut, M. A., Zonderman, A. B., & Davatzikos, C. (2003). Longitudinal magnetic resonance imaging studies of older adults: a shrinking brain. *Journal of Neuroscience, 23*(8), 3295-3301.

Rhee, C., & Gatz, M. (1993). Cross-generational attributions concerning locus of control beliefs. *International Journal of Aging and Human Development, 37*(2), 153-161.

Rikli, R. E., & Edwards, D. J. (1991). Effects of a three-year exercise program on motor function and cognitive processing speed in older women. *Research Quarterly for Exercise and Sports, 62*(1), 61-67.

Roberts, B. W., & Caspi, A. (2003). The cumulative continuity model of personality development: Striking a balance between continuity and change in personality traits across the life course. In U. M. Staudinger & U. Lindenberger (Eds.), *Understanding human development: dialogues with lifespan psychology* (pp. 183-214). Boston: Kluwer.

Roberts, B. W., & DelVecchio, W. F. (2000). The rank-order consistency of personality from childhood to old age: A quantitative review of longitudinal studies. *Psychological Bulletin, 126*, 3-25.

Ross, C. E., & Mirowsky, J. (2002). Age and the gender gap in the sense of personal control. *Social Psychology Quarterly, 65*(2), 125-145.

Ruch-Monachon, M., Perrig-Chiello, P., & Staehelin, H. B. (1999). Persönlichkeit. In P. Perrig-Chiello, H. B. Staehelin & W. J. Perrig (Eds.), *Wohlbefinden, Gesundheit und kognitive Kompetenz im Alter* (pp. 105-108). Bern: Haupt.

Rupprecht, R., Gunzelmann, T., Oswald, W. D., Lang, E., Baumann, H., & Stosberg, M. (1993). Bedingungen der Erhaltung und Förderung von Selbständigkeit im höheren Lebens-Alter (SIMA) - Teil II: Methoden der Bedingungsanalyse und Trainingsevaluation. *Zeitschrift für Gerontopsychologie und -psychiatrie, 6*, 217-227.

Ryff, C. D. (1989). Happiness is everything, or is it? explorations on the meaning of psychological well-being. *Journal of Personality and Social Psychology, 57*(6), 1069-1081.

Salthouse, T. A. (1996). The processing-speed theory of adult age differences in cognition. *Psychological Review, 103*(3), 403-428.

Schacter, D. L. (1987). Implicit memory: history and current status. *Journal of Experimental Psychology: Learning, Memory, and Cognition, 13*, 501-518.

Schilling, O. K. (2005). Cohort- and age-related decline in elder's life satisfaction: is there really a paradox? *European Journal of Ageing, 2*, 254-263.

Schmader, T., & Johns, M. (2003). Converging evidence that stereotype threat reduces working memory capacity. *Journal of Personality and Social Psychology, 85*(3), 440-452.

Schneider, W., Eschman, A., & Zuccolotto, A. (2002). *E-Prime user's guide*. Pittsburgh: Psychology Software Inc.

Scogin, F., & Bienias, J. L. (1988). A three-year follow-up of older adult participants in a memory-skills training program. *Psychology and Aging, 3*(4), 334-337.

Scogin, F., Storandt, M., & Lott, L. (1985). Memory-skills training, memory complaints, and depression in older adults. *Journal of Gerontology, 40*(5), 562-568.

Scuffham, P., Chaplin, S., & Legood, R. (2003). Incidence and costs of unintentional falls in older people in the United Kingdom. *Journal of Epidemiology and Community Health, 57*, 740-744.

Singh, N. A., Clements, K. M., & Fiatarone, M. A. (1997). A randomized controlled trial of progressive resistance training in depressed elderly. *Journal of Gerontology: Medical Sciences, 52A*(1), M27-M35.

Smith, J. (2003). The gain-loss dynamic in lifespan development: Implications for change in self and personality during old and very old age. In U. M. Staudinger & U. Lindenberger (Eds.), *Understanding human development: dialogues with lifespan psychology* (pp. 215-241). Boston: Kluwer.

Smith, J., & Baltes, P. B. (1996). Altern aus psychologischer Perspektive: Trends und Profile im hohen Alter. In K. U. Mayer & P. B. Baltes (Eds.), *Die Berliner Altersstudie*. Berlin: Akademie-Verlag.

Smith, J., Borchelt, M., Maier, H., & Jopp, D. (2002). Health and well-being in the young old and oldest old. *Journal of Social Issues, 58*(4), 715-732.

Smith, J., Fleeson, W., Geiselmann, B., Settersten, R., & Kunzmann, U. (1996). Wohlbefinden im hohen Alter: Vorhersagen aufgrund objektiver Lebensbedingungen und subjektiver Bewertung. In K. U. Mayer & P. B. Baltes (Eds.), *Die Berliner Altersstudie* (pp. 497-523). Berlin: Akademia Verlag.

Spirduso, W. W., & Cronin, D. L. (2001). Exercise dose-response effects on quality of life and independent living in older adults. *Medicine and Science in Sports and Exercise, 33*(6), S598-S608.

Staudinger, U. M., Freund, A. M., Linden, M., & Maas, I. (1996a). Selbst, Persönlichkeit und Lebensgestaltung im Alter. In K. U. Mayer & P. B. Baltes (Eds.), *Die Berliner Altersstudie* (pp. 321-350). Berlin: Akademie Verlag.

Staudinger, U. M., Freund, A. M., Linden, M., & Maas, I. (1996b). Selbst, Persönlichkeit und Lebensgestaltung im Alter: Psychologische Widerstandsfähigkeit und Vulnerabilität. In K. U. Mayer & P. B. Baltes (Eds.), *Die Berliner Altersstudie* (pp. 321-350). Berlin: Akademie Verlag.

Stein, R., Blanchard-Fields, F., & Hertzog, C. (2002). The effects of age-stereotype priming on the memory performance of older adults. *Experimental Aging Research, 28*(2), 169-181.

Steinhagen-Thiessen, E., & Borchelt, M. (1996). Morbidität, Medikation und Funktionalität im Alter. In K. U. Mayer & P. B. Baltes (Eds.), *Die Berliner Altersstudie*. Berlin: Akademie-Verlag.

Stewart, A. L., & King, A. C. (1991). Evaluation the efficacy of physical activity for influencing quality of life outcomes in older adults. *Annals of Behavioral Medicine, 13*, 108-116.

Stigsdotter, A., & Bäckman, L. (1989). Comparisons of different forms of memory training in old age. In M. A. Luszcz & T. Nettlebeck (Eds.), *Psychological development: Perspectives across the life span*. Amsterdam: Elsevier.

Stigsdotter Neely, A., & Bäckman, L. (1995). Effects of multifactorial memory training in old age: generalizability across tasks and individuals. *Journals of Gerontology B: Psychological Sciences and Social Sciences, 50*(3), P134-140.

Stones, M. J., & Kozma, A. (1996). Activity, exercise, and behavior. In J. E. Birren & K. W. Schaie (Eds.), *Handbook of the psychology of aging* (4 ed., pp. 338-352). San Diego: Academic Press.

Strayer, D., Wickens, C., & Braune, R. (1987). Adult age differences in the speed and capacity of information processing. *Psychology and Aging, 2*, 99-110.

Stuck, A. (2003). Sturzprävention und Gesundheitsförderung im Alter: Multidimensionales geriatrisches Assessment. Referat an der Arbeitstagung "Osteoporose und Stürze im Alter – Fakten und Handlungsbedarf" vom 4. und 5. September in Bern. Retrieved March 1st, 2007, from http://www.bag.admin.ch/themen/medizin/00683/01988/01994/index.html?lang=de

Sugarman, L. (2001). *Life-span development: frameworks, accounts and strategies* (2 ed.). Hove: Psychology Press.

Swiss Federal Office of Statistics. (2005). *Statistisches Jahrbuch der Schweiz 2005*. Zürich: Verlag Neue Zürcher Zeitung.

Tellegen, A., Lykken, D., Bouchard, T. J., Wilcox, K. J., Segal, N. L., & Rich, S. (1988). Personality similarity in twins reared apart and together. *Journal of Personality and Social Psychology, 54*, 1031-1039.

Tewes, U. (Ed.). (2001). *Hamburg-Wechsler Intelligenztest für Erwachsene, Revision 1991*. Bern: Hans Huber.

Tomporowski, P. D., & Ellis, N. R. (1986). Effects of exercise on cognitive processes: A review. *Psychological Bulletin, 99*(3), 338-346.

Touron, D. R., & Hertzog, C. (2004). Distinguishing age differences in knowledge, strategy use, and confidence during strategic skill acquisition. *Psychology and Aging, 19*(3), 452-466.

Tranel, D., & Damasio, A. R. (2002). Neurobiological foundations of human memory. In A. Baddeley, M. D. Kopelman & B. A. Wilson (Eds.), *The handbook of memory disorders* (2nd ed.). West Sussex: John Wiley and Sons.

Verhaeghen, P., Marcoen, A., & Goossens, L. (1992). Improving memory performance in the aged through mnemonic training: a meta-analytic study. *Psychology and Aging, 7*(2), 242-251.

Voelcker-Rehage, C., Godde, B., & Staudinger, U. M. (2006). Bewegung, körperliche und geistige Mobilität im Alter. *Bundesgesundheitsblatt-Gesundheitsforschung-Gesundheitsschutz, 49*, 558-566.

Wallhagen, M. I., Strawbridge, W. J., Kaplan, G. A., & Cohen, R. D. (1994). Impact of internal health locus of control on health outcomes for older men and women: A longitudinal perspective. *Gerontologist, 34*(3), 299-306.

Walter, U., Schneider, N., & Bisson, S. (2006). Krankheitslast und Gesundheit im Alter. *Bundesgesundheitsblatt-Gesundheitsforschung-Gesundheitsschutz, 49*, 537-546.

Williams, P., & Lord, S. R. (1997). Effects of group exercise on cognitive functioning and mood in older women. *Australian and New Zealand Journal of Public Health, 21*(1), 45-52.

Willis, M. W., Ketter, T. A., Kimbrell, T. A., George, M. S., Herscovitch, P., Danielson, A. L., et al. (2002). Age, sex and laterality effects on cerebral glucose metabolism in healthy adults. *Psychiatry Research, 114*(1), 23-37.

Wilson, J. F. (2004). Frailty - and its dangerous effects - might be preventable. *Annals of Internal Medicine, 141*, 489-492.

Wolinsky, F. D., Wyrwich, K. W., Babu, A. N., Kroenke, K., & Tierney, W. M. (2003). Age, aging, and the sense of control among older adults: A longitudinal reconsideration. *Journal of Gerontology, 58B*(4), 212-220.

Wolters, G., Theunissen, I., Bemelmans, K. J., van der Does, A. J. W., & Spinhoven, P. (1996). Immediate and intermediate-term effectiveness of a memory training program for the elderly. *Journal of Cognitive Rehabilitation, 14*(3), 16-22.

World Health Organization. (2007). *The ICD-10 classification of mental and behavioural disorders. Clinical descriptions and diagnostic guidelines.* Geneva: World Health Organisation.

Yesavage, J. A., Rose, T. L., & Spiegel, D. (1982). Relaxation training and memory improvement in elderly normals: Correlation of anxiety rating and recall improvement. *Experimental Aging Research, 8*, 195-198.

Yesavage, J. A., Sheikh, J. I., Friedman, L., & Tanke, E. (1990). Learning mnemonics: Roles of aging and subtle cognitive impairment. *Psychology and Aging, 5*, 133-137.

# APPENDIX I

| Session | Semantic activ. (SA) | Stereotypes | Working memory | Theory | Voluntary homework / "fun"** |
|---|---|---|---|---|---|
| 1 | | INTRODUCTION<br>Welcome, overview of training, goals, introduction of coaches und fellow participants | | | | |
| 2 | | Baseline assessement<br>word list, word fluency, getting acquainted with the computer (flower task), how to remember each other's names | | | | |
| 3 | SA 1 | Reaction time task | Flower* | Attention and concentration | photo stories, chains of terms, Mikado, translation errors |
| 4 | SA 2 | Reaction time task | Flower* | A model of memory | intruder, opposites, follow the lines, scale |
| 5 | SA 3 | Reaction time task | Senso | Sensory memory | "Stecker", chains of terms, allocation |
| 6 | | Assessment 1<br>1. word list (5-10min), 2. Fluency (8min), 3. semantic activation (SA 4, 5min), 4. fun (5min), 5. working-memory training (3min), 6. Delayed recall (2min), 7. Lexical decision (4min). | | | | |
| 7 | SA 5 | Lexical decision | Senso | Visual perception | Optical illusions |
| 8 | SA 6 | Lexical decision | Senso | Hearing | identify sounds |
| 9 | SA 7 | Lexical decision | Senso | Sense of smell | identify smells |
| 10 | | Practice Session (no theory)<br>Semantic activation (SA 8, 6min), introduction C&D task (15min), Fun (10min), Reaction time task (6min) | | | | |
| 11 | SA 9 | Reaction time task | C&D | Sense of touch | identify objects by sense of touch |
| 12 | SA 10 | Reaction time task | C&D | The preferred sense | „Stecker", chains of terms, wanted: animal friends |
| 13 | SA 11 | Reaction time task | C&D | Short-term memory | Guild signs, allocation, stamps |
| 14 | | Assessment 2<br>1. word list (5-10min), 2. Fluency (8min), 3. semantic activation (SA 12, 5min), 4. fun (5min), 5. working-memory training (C&D, 3min), 6. Delayed recall (2min), 7. Lexical decision (4min). | | | | |
| 15 | SA 13 | Lexical decision | C&D | Long-term memory | Setting a table, analogies, proverbs |
| 16 | SA 14 | Lexical decision | C&D | Repetition of the model of memory | Criminal, proverbs, spaghetti-reading |
| 17 | SA 15 | Lexical decision | Senso | External influences on memory | „Stecker", translation errors, hands |
| 18 | SA 16 | Reaction time task | Animal Span | | Presentation about age influences on cognition (guest speaker Prof. Perrig) | |
| 19 | SA 17 | Reaction time task | Animal Span | Systematical reconstruction | delete and add, geo-sheep, overlapping circles |
| 20 | SA 18 | Reaction time task | Animal Span | Automating as memory aid | Wanted (fairy tales), anagrams, wheel of fortune |
| 21 | SA 19 | Reaction time task | Animal Span | External memory aids | proverbs, figures, classification |
| 22 | | Assessment 3<br>1. word list (5-10min), 2. Fluency (8min), 3. semantic activation (5min), 4. fun (5min), 5. working-memory training (Animal Span, 3min), 6. Delayed recall (2min), 7. Lexical decision (4min). | | | | |
| 23 | | **Presentation of first training results, good-bye** | | | | |

\* *The flower task is not a working memory task, instead it served to familiarize participants with the computer*
\*\**some of the fun exercises are described in more detail in appendix 3*
Note: *The sessions always started with semantic activation, followed by Stereotypes and working memory training, followed by a second round of Stereotypes, working memory and semantic activation.*

# APPENDIX II

| Session | Topic | Content |
|---|---|---|
| 1 | *no theory* | -- |
| 2 | Remembering names | Participants learned to combine/connect another persons name with a funny picture to remember it better (e.g. Herr Hoppeler hopping like a bunny), or to repeat a name or to use it right away. |
| 3 | Attention and concentration | It was stressed that attention is crucial for remembering, and that older people are more easily distracted. Tipps were given how to limit distractions. |
| 4 | A model of memory | A model of memory was introduced containing „sensual memory", short-term memory, and long-term memory. This structure would serve as basis for further sessions. |
| 5 | Sensory memory | How long can information be stored in the sensual memory? What is the function of this storage? How is it affected by aging? |
| 6 | *no theory* | -- |
| 7 | Perception (visual) | It was shown that our perceptions are not always correct reflections of reality. How do expectations influence perceptions? Presentation of optical illusions. |
| 8 | Hearing | Anatomical structure of the ear / how do we hear / what happens to the ear and hearing in old age/ Exercise: Identification of sounds (e.g. Boat, chickens, train etc.) |
| 9 | Smell | Informations about the human sense of smell, scents/odours and memory. Identification of different smells |
| 10 | *no theory* | -- |

| 11 | Sense of touch | Functions of the skin / why do we need a sense of touch / Exercise: Identification of different objects only by sense of touch (e.g. onion, teabag, syringe etc.) |
|---|---|---|
| 12 | The preferred sense | Which is my preferred sense? Am I an auditive, visual or tactile type? How can I use that knowledge to my advantage? |
| 13 | Short-term memory | How is information transferred from sensual memory into short-term memory? Function of short-term memory / How much information can be stored? / what is chunking? (Chunking was only mentioned, *not* practised!) |
| 14 | *no theory* | -- |
| 15 | Long-term memory | How does information get into long.term memory? What is the function of long-term memory? What happens in the brain when information is stored? Age effects on long-term memory |
| 16 | Repetition of the model of memory | A repetition of the memory model from session 4, integration of the knowledge acquired in the last seesions into this model, exercise: matching of terms to different components of memory. |
| 17 | External influences on memory | Influence of nutrition and exercise on memory / influence of biological rhythm („inner clock") |
| 18 | Presentation about age influences on cognition (guest speaker Prof. Perrig) | Professor Perrig presented results from different studies about aging and cognition / which parts of cognition are affected by aging? |
| 19 | Systematical reconstruction | Systematical reconstruction as help with retrieval problems in memory, or „how to search" |
| 20 | Automating as memory aid | How automating can reduce memory load / how automate an action |
| 21 | External memory aids | What external memory aids exist? How to use them, when to use them |
| 22 | *no theory* | -- |
| 23 | Presentation of first training results | e.g. how many items could be remembered in the cats and dogs task now in comparison to the first few sessions? How much faster were the reactions in the reaction time task? |

# APPENDIX III

**Examples of voluntary homework**

Examples of exercises:

*„Wanted"*: Participants were given four or five sentences which described a character or an object without mentioning its name. They then had to find out which character/object fitted the descriptions. Examples were characters of fairy tales, or a specific animal.

*„Proverbs"*: A square was presented consisting of the scrambled letters of a popular saying. Participants first had to find the starting letter. The next letter would then be found in adjacent position (left, right, up or down, not diagonally), the one after that again adjacent to the last letter, and so on, until the saying formed one continuous line using up all the letters of the square.

*„Setting a table"*: Participants were given a picture of a table set for several people with cutlery, glasses etc. for several courses. However, some spoons, glasses or knives were missing. Participants had to find these missing objects.

*„Word-tumble"*: Participants were given one word with about ten letters and then had to make as many new words as possible out of these letters. Only the letters contained in the original words could be used, and each letter only once. The new words could be of any length shorter than eleven letters.

*„Guild signs"*: A sheet with several guild signs was handed out, and the participants had to guess which sign belonged to which guild. The same task was repeated later with objects found in fairy tales.

*„Allocation"*: Participants were given a grid containing several objects. The task was to find out the rule according to which the objects had been placed in the grid and then place a few other objects in the proper fields.

*„Mikado"*: Participants were given a picture of Mikado sticks tossed in a pile. They had to find out in which order one had to lift off the single sticks so as not to disturb the remaining sticks.

*„Analogies"*: Participants had to complete analogies like the follwing: „A head to the body is like a blossom to the ......". The correct answer in this case would be stem, as a blossom stands in the same relation to ist stem as the head of a person to the body.

Ideas for these exercises were taken from different sources (Fischer, Lehrl, & Grässel, 2002; Fischer, Lehrl, & Kindl, 1998; Fischer, Lehrl, & Wurzer, 1992, 1993, 1997; Klauer, 2002; Oswald, 1998).

## ACKNOWLEDGMENTS

First of all, I'd like to thank Professor Pasqualina Perrig-Chiello for all the time, work, and enthusiasm she invested in this dissertation. It was always very motivating and intellectually stimulating to talk to her about the project, and her suggestions have improved this thesis enormously.

I'd also like to thank Professor Walter Perrig for giving me the opportunity to participate in the ExTrA project, and for believing that I was "doctor material". His many helpful comments have contributed significantly to this project.

The ExTrA project was a collaboration of many people; I'd especially like to thank Dr. Martin Buschkühl for his collaboration on the cognitive training, as well as the whole team from the Institute of Anatomy.

This study would not have been possible without our wonderful participants. I truly had a great time working with them, and they have taught me more than they will ever know. A heartfelt "thank you" goes to all of them.

I would not be who I am today without the continuing love and support from my parents. They were there for me every step of the way and have always believed in me. Thank you for always being there for me.

Last but not least, I'd like to thank my husband John. He has been with me in this project from the start and has experienced all the ups and downs with me. I don't know what I would do without his love, support and encouragement. I really cannot thank him enough.

And finally, I'd like to thank my daughter Ariel for putting everything into perspective, and for giving me every reason to finish this dissertation.

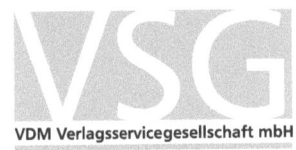

Die VDM Verlagsservicegesellschaft sucht für wissenschaftliche Verlage abgeschlossene und herausragende

## Dissertationen, Habilitationen, Diplomarbeiten, Master Theses, Magisterarbeiten usw.

für die kostenlose Publikation als Fachbuch.

Sie verfügen über eine Arbeit, die hohen inhaltlichen und formalen Ansprüchen genügt, und haben Interesse an einer honorarvergüteten Publikation?

Dann senden Sie bitte erste Informationen über sich und Ihre Arbeit per Email an *info@vdm-vsg.de*.

**Sie erhalten kurzfristig unser Feedback!**

VDM Verlagsservicegesellschaft mbH
Dudweiler Landstr. 99　　　　　　Telefon　+49 681 3720 174
D - 66123 Saarbrücken　　　　　　Fax　　　+49 681 3720 1749
**www.vdm-vsg.de**

Die VDM Verlagsservicegesellschaft mbH vertritt

  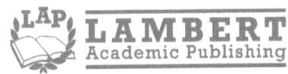  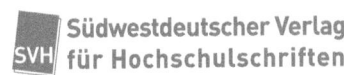

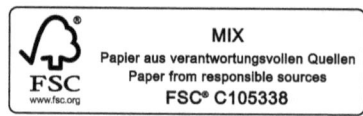

Printed by Books on Demand GmbH, Norderstedt / Germany